SKIN, THE HAIR & NAILS

THE SKIN, HAIR & NAILS

The Reader's Digest Association, Inc.

Pleasantville, New York

London New York Sydney Montreal

The Skin, Hair and Nails

was created and produced by
Carroll & Brown Limited
20 Lonsdale Road
London NW6 6RD
for Reader's Digest, London

Library of Congress Cataloging-in-Publication Data
The skin, hair, and nails : your body, your health /
Readers Digest.—1st ed.
  p. cm.
  ISBN 0-7621-0484-8 (Hardcover)
1. Skin—Popular works. 2. Hair—Popular works. 3. Nails
(Anatomy)--Popular works. I. Reader's Digest
Association.
  RL87.S56 2003
  616.5--dc21

                                    2003008603

The information in this book is for reference only; it is not intended as a substitute for a doctor's diagnosis and care. The editors urge anyone with continuing medical problems or symptoms to consult a doctor.

American Edition Produced by
NOVA Graphic Services, Inc.
2370 York Road, Suite A9A
Jamison, PA 18929 USA
(215) 542-3900

President
David Davenport

Editorial Director
Robin C Bonner

Composition Manager
Steve Magnin

Associate Project Editor
Linnea Hermanson

Otolaryngology Specialist Consultant
Dr Milan Amin, MD
Drexel University College of Medicine/Hahneman Medical College, Philadelphia

CONTRIBUTORS
Wynnie Chan, BSc, PhD, Public Health Nutritionist

Dr Sandeep H Cliff, MB, BSc, MRCP, Consultant Dermatologist,
Honorary Senior Lecturer, Surrey

Mr Brian Coghlan, MD, FRCS (Plast), Consultant Plastic Surgeon, Guy's Hospital, London

F J Cunningham, MRIPH MIT (Lond), Member of the Institute of Trichologists,
The Trichology Centre, Rochdale

Christel Edwards-de Graauw, Nail Technician, Nail Artist and Makeup Artist,
Fingernails Direct, Northern Ireland

Dr Colin Fleming, BSc, MB ChB, MRCP,
Consultant Dermatologist, Department of Dermatology, Ninewells Hospital, Dundee,
Honorary Senior Lecturer, University of Dundee

Katy Glynne, BSc, MRPharmS, Dip Pharmacy Practice,
Clinical Services Manager, Charing Cross Hospital, London,
Clinical Lecturer, The School of Pharmacy, University of London

Dr Lesley Hickin, MB BS, BSc, DRCOG, MRCGP, General Practitioner

Dr Shona Ogilvie, MB ChB, MRCGP, Clinical Fellow,
University Department of Dermatology, Ninewells Hospital, Dundee

Penny Preston, MB ChB, MRGCP, Medical Writer

Beverly Westwood, RN, BSc, MSc, Research Director to Mr Brian Coghlan

For Reader's Digest
Editor in Chief and Publishing Director Neil E Wertheimer
Managing Editor Suzanne G Beason
Art Director Michele Laseau
Production Technology Manager Douglas A Croll
Manufacturing Manager John L Cassidy
Production Coordinator Leslie Ann Caraballo

The Skin, Hair and Nails

Awareness of health issues and expectations of medicine are greater today than ever before. A long and healthy life has come to be looked on as not so much a matter of luck but as almost a right. However, as our knowledge of health and the causes of disease has grown, it has become increasingly clear that health is something that we can all influence, for better or worse, through choices we make in our lives. *Your Body Your Health* is designed to help you make the right choices to make the most of your health potential. Each volume in the series focuses on a different physiological system of the body, explaining what it does and how it works. There is a wealth of advice and health tips on diet, exercise and lifestyle factors, as well as the health checks you can expect throughout life. You will find out what can go wrong and what can be done about it, and learn from people's real-life experiences of diagnosis and treatment. Finally, there is a detailed A to Z index of the major conditions which can affect the system. The series builds into a complete user's manual for the care and maintenance of the entire body.

This volume examines the body's largest organ, demonstrating how the skin keeps out the hostile world and protects our internal organs. Follow the fascinating life story of skin and hair cells, and how they respond to our bodies' aging processes. Find out how a single cell detects a featherlight touch, how the skin and hair get their color, and why we need nails. By monitoring what is normal for your skin and hair you can gain an understanding of what threatens them, and use our guides to devise basic care routines for the skin, hair and nails to make sure yours always look their best. Discover how important diet is for the health of skin, hair and nails, and how to ensure you get all the nutrients they need. The sun is one of the biggest threats your skin must face, so here are sensible guidelines on safety in the sun. Finally, you can read what can go wrong with the skin, who are the professionals involved in diagnosing and treating skin problems, and how drugs, light and revolutionary surgical techniques can help to put them right.

Contents

1

How your skin, hair, and nails work

2

Keeping your skin, hair, and nails healthy

3

What happens when things go wrong

The life story of the skin

Despite the almost universal human preoccupation with appearance, most of us do not realize that our bodies have ingenious and sophisticated features that really are just skin deep. Evolution has given us a highly specialized organ—the skin—that puts us in touch with the outside world while protecting the delicate organs inside the body from potential dangers in our environment.

The skin is the largest organ in the body, and it fulfils many vital functions. It forms a protective barrier between the body and the environment and plays an important role in the immune system by detecting infections. It helps regulate the body's temperature, stopping us from overheating (by sweating), and it protects us from damage from ultraviolet (UV) radiation. As a sensory organ, the skin helps us discern conditions in the outside world—temperature, texture, vibrations—and is a medium for social and sexual communication.

A failure in any one of these functions can have serious consequences. If temperature regulation fails, we can develop heat stroke or hypothermia. If the barrier function is affected, we can lose fluid and become dehydrated. Sensory incapacity can result in physical injury, from burns to bruises, and a failure of the immune response can lead to overwhelming infection. Furthermore, because of the skin's importance to our appearance and self-esteem, skin problems often have a social and psychological impact in addition to their medical consequences. In fact, many people with a skin problem that is not seriously harmful physically still find their lives blighted by real or perceived rejection by society.

HOW SKIN EVOLVED

Millions of years of evolutionary development were needed to produce the naked human beings we are today, with skin, hair, and nails that seemingly function primarily as aids to beauty and sexual attraction. The skin is

On average, every square inch of skin contains 60 hairs, 90 sebaceous glands, 625 sweat glands, 19 feet of blood vessels, and 19,000 sensory cells.

composed of tightly packed cells arranged in two layers: the epidermis (top layer) and the dermis (lower layer). Melanocytes—specialized cells in the epidermis—give skin (and hair) its color, but the principal role of these cells is to protect the delicate DNA in the cell nucleus from damage by ultraviolet radiation. This evolutionary step was essential once humans started to become less hairy.

WHY WE NEED HAIR

In most mammals, hair or fur plays an essential role in survival, particularly in heat conservation. This is not the case in humans. Scalp hair does function as a protection against cold, minor injuries, and the cancer-inducing effects of UV radiation, but its main role in human society is as an organ of display to attract a mate—hence its importance to the cosmetics industry.

HOW THE SKIN DEVELOPS

The skin, hair, and nails develop early in the life of the embryo: The basal layer of the epidermis begins to develop just four weeks after conception. By seven weeks, flat cells overlying the basal layer form the periderm, which is cast

Different skin colors and hues

Skin color results from the amount of the pigment melanin that is in your skin. People with darker skins have greater amounts of melanin in their skin; this provides more protection against the damaging effects of sunshine.

off at about 24 weeks and replaced by the more complicated double-layered structure of the epidermis and dermis. The function of the periderm is not wholly understood, but it is probably concerned with the absorption of nutrients.

Nails start to take shape 10 weeks after conception. The dermis (mesoderm) develops at 11 weeks, and by 12 weeks, indented basal buds of the epidermis form the hair bulbs, with dermal papillae supplying vessels and nerves to the epidermal structures. By 17 weeks, fingerprint ridges are determined and sebaceous glands are becoming active under the influence of maternal hormones that cross the placenta. This sebaceous activity continues until a baby is about six months old, then it tapers off and doesn't kick in again until hormones become active at puberty.

The teens are often a bad time for skin, but problems are not inevitable and can certainly be treated. Adult skin reflects general health and social behavior. Anyone who wants his or her skin to remain relatively soft and unwrinkled until late in life needs to take some precautions: It is vital to avoid excess sun exposure and not to smoke. Ultraviolet light is the cause of almost all the visible changes in sun-exposed areas such as the face and the backs of the hands. Sunblock offers partial but not complete protection.

Keeping the skin clean is important to prevent infection and odor, but excess washing can cause dry skin. Washing with harsh soaps strips the skin surface of its natural oils, so it's best to choose products with care and avoid having your hands in water for long periods of time. Similarly, excess washing, color treating, and perming rob the hair of protective oil.

KERATIN: WONDER MATERIAL

The basic protein that makes up the skin, hair, and nails is keratin, an amazing substance that forms the major part of the skin and hair and 98 percent of the nail plate. Keratin is also found in many other animal species: Its toughness and flexibility make it the perfect building block

Skin, hair, and nail formation
After 5 months of development, a fetus has sweat glands, fine hair on its head, and fully formed eyelids, fingernails, and toenails.

PROTECTION FOR LIFE

The resilience of our skin, hair, and nails is amazing. For most of us, just a little effort in terms of daily maintenance, protection, and a good balanced diet will repay us with a lifetime of healthy skin, hair, and nails.

BABY

CHILDHOOD

Tender care
A baby's skin is thinner, more fragile, and less oily than an adult's. To protect its skin, use baby lotion to seal in moisture after a bath.

Oopsie daisy!
Children regularly fall down, scraping or cutting their skin. At this age, the skin heals quickly, but a little antiseptic cream can help prevent infection.

to ensure that birds' feathers fly and that horses' hooves are hard. Keratin not only forms the tough substance of the cells, but it also creates the anchoring pegs that hold the cells together, side by side and layer upon layer.

There are many different types of keratin in different species and body parts, but they are all made from the same basic amino acid building blocks of cysteine, arginine, lysine, and histidine. Cysteine provides the sulfur cross-bonds that link some types of keratin together. These are the bonds that are split by heat or chemicals when a permanent wave is applied to the hair (the bonds reform after the hair cools or the chemicals are neutralized).

The gene sequences that make the different types of keratin have been revealed through research on people in whom keratin production has gone wrong. Some of the most important and life-threatening skin diseases occur when keratin formation is disturbed. Disorders of keratin formation can disrupt the basic structure of the skin: They can make layers of skin slide over each other and let in fluid, causing severe blistering and subsequent infection. Today, skin biopsies can be taken from fetuses known to be at risk of inheriting severe genetic skin disorders—such as Netherton's syndrome and epidermolysis bullosa—at around 16 weeks development.

From boys to men
Teenage boys start to develop facial hair and their skin becomes more oily. In time, they will all need to start shaving, but every male develops different amounts of body hair.

Sun protection
It is extremely important to protect your skin from sun exposure. Wearing sunscreen, sunglasses, and a wide-brimmed hat will help prevent the aging effects of UV radiation.

TEENAGE

ADULT

ELDERLY

Keeping skin supple
When stubble is shaved, the skin is stripped of its natural oils. After shaving, moisturize your skin to prevent dryness.

Foot work
The skin on your feet should receive regular attention. Elderly people often find that their mobility is enhanced by podiatrist treatment.

The majority of skin diseases are not life-threatening but instead tend to linger throughout life. Problems such as eczema and psoriasis make up a large proportion of the skin disorders that drive us to seek medical help.

KEEPING UP APPEARANCES

A person's physical appearance is the first thing we notice about him or her in social situations: 80 percent of our memory of a person comes from the face—far more than from the voice, and only a minimal amount comes from the content of the conversation. It is no wonder, therefore, that so many of us spend a lot of our time, money, and

effort to make ourselves as attractive as possible to others. In humans, the face has evolved to become the most important visual tool, with more than 30 separate muscles involved in controlling facial expression.

Beauty is also a visual impression of form and color. Appreciation of beauty is subjective, but in any one society, there is usually broad agreement on those features that are more—and less—attractive. In modern society, large numbers of people are prepared to spend time and money and even to undergo considerable pain and discomfort in pursuit of the cultural "ideal" of beauty.

In the 20th century, the cosmetics industry grew to a multi-billion-dollar global concern, but efforts to alter appearance are nothing new. There is evidence of makeup being used in civilizations dating back into antiquity, and tattooing, scarification (deliberately scarring the body), and piercing have been practiced in cultures all over the world for thousands of years. The arts of tattooing and piercing traditionally had limited appeal in the West, but they are becoming increasingly popular among groups from all social and economic strata.

Fashions in body adornment constantly shift. At various times in history, wigs have been the height of fashion, but at others close-cropped hair has been preferred. Hair color, length, and degree of curl also drift in and out of favor. One of the earliest uses of makeup was to make warriors more fearsome to their opponents, but it soon became a way to enhance attractiveness. It has been used to produce the "pale and interesting" look considered desirable in much of the past, but this has given way to the era of the suntan—still with us despite increasing evidence of its harmful effects on the skin.

Identity art
Throughout history, skin decoration and body art have been of deep significance in cultures around the world. They have been used to provide a link to ancestors, to convey religious symbolism, to mark rites of passage, and to emphasize visual characteristics.

SKIN COLOR

A number of factors influence skin color. Genetics plays a major part, as do geographical region and the amount of time spent outdoors. Other factors include hemoglobin, internally produced pigments such as bilirubin, and the amounts of melanin and pheomelanin in the skin and hair. In many conditions, temporary or permanent changes to skin and hair color, which may lead to distress and even psychological illness, can occur.

Skin color can be a major factor in all sorts of prejudices, and not just between races of different color. Departures from the norm in a society can have unhappy consequences for individuals and their place within society.

SKIN IN THE FUTURE

The global loss of protective ozone over the past 20 years means that we are being exposed to more UV radiation than were previous generations, even though most of us are more "sun aware." UV damage initially causes fine lines on the skin, but repeated sun exposure eventually makes deep wrinkles and may result in skin cancer. Estimates suggest that a 1 percent decrease in ozone can result in a 5 percent increase in skin cancer rates: Ozone depletion may increase our children's risk of skin cancer by up to 15 percent, making vigilance in skin protection vital.

On a more positive note for the future, scientists have succeeded in culturing epidermal skin from a tiny undamaged area of human skin. This has major implications for severe burns victims, greatly increasing their chances of survival and minimizing eventual scarring. Parallel to this has been the development of artificial skin, a nonliving material free from bacteria and viruses. Artificial skin is used to support the grafted epidermis, which then regenerates the

Sample of artificial skin
Scientific advances have led to the development of artificially grown skin. Its three layers—epidermis, dermis, and hypodermis—have all the specialized cells and structures found in normal skin.

dermal layer. The world's first factory making human skin opened in 1995. Researchers are also looking at the genetics involved in baldness and graying hair with the intent to modify the genes responsible in order to prevent both processes. In the not too distant future, gene therapy may also be the key to successful treatment of melanoma.

*There are reputed to be more than 2000 skin conditions,
but two thirds of skin diseases are caused by fewer than 10 conditions.
More than 65 million Americans per year visit a doctor
for skin problems, including skin cancer.*

1

How your skin, hair, and nails work

Your amazing skin, hair, and nails

Your skin is the largest and most versatile system of tissue organization that you have. As a barrier between you and the outside world, it fulfills many roles, starting with keeping water out and your insides safely covered.

WHY DO WE NEED SKIN?

The skin—the outer covering of the body—has several extremely important functions. It protects you from water loss and damage from ultraviolet radiation. It helps you regulate your body temperature. It is an effective barrier against injury and invading microorganisms, and it is involved in the immune response that protects the body from foreign substances that do manage to penetrate it. Nerve impulses from the skin communicate sensation to the brain. The skin plays an essential part in the production of vitamin D—vital for healthy bones. In addition, it has a role in display and sexual attraction.

THE CHANGING FACE OF SKIN

Although the basic structure of the skin is the same over the entire body, there are local variations linked to differences in function. For example, the skin on the palms of the hands and soles of the feet has no hair and is much thicker than in other areas in order to toughen it up. Skin regularly exposed to sunlight is darker than skin hidden from view to help protect it from ultraviolet radiation.

The appearance of the skin varies throughout life, and even day-to-day changes can occur, depending on your emotions and state of well-being: Skin abnormalities can often be the first warning of internal illness.

The skin is the largest organ in the body, weighing on average 9 pounds and covering a surface area of about 2.5 square yards.

There are two types of hairs on your body: short, fine vellus hairs and longer, thicker terminal hairs. Turn to pages 30–31 to check out their differences—and find out why some vellus hairs turn into terminal hairs at puberty.

Your nails protect protect the sensitive tips of your fingers and toes from damage, and they also serve as valuable tools for tasks involving prying or scratching. Pages 32–33 take a close-up look at these appendages.

Tiny blood vessels in the dermis not only nourish the skin and help fight infection by bringing in white blood cells; they also help the body cool off or warm up as required. Pages 26–27 describe how.

How your skin, hair, and nails work

Hair, nails, and glands
Parts of your epidermis have become specialized and form the so-called epidermal appendages, which project deep into the dermis. These are the hairs and nails, the sebaceous glands, and the sweat glands.

A sweat gland *is a long, coiled, hollow tube that transports sweat to the skin's surface so it can evaporate. To find out more about how the body stays cool, turn to pages 26–27.*

Each strand of hair *extends .16–.20 in. into the skin's subterranean layers. To find out more, see pages 30–31.*

The epidermis *is the outermost layer of the skin. The dead skin cells are continually shed and replaced from the cell layers beneath. Find out how and why this happens on pages 18–19.*

Sensory nerve endings *in the dermis provide you with your sense of touch—one of the five key senses. Find out more on pages 22–23.*

A sebaceous gland *produces sebum, which lubricates, protects, and waterproofs the skin. Find out more about this wonder fluid on pages 24–25.*

The dermis *is the layer of connective tissue beneath the epidermis that forms the bulk of the skin. Discover more about its crucial supporting role on pages 20–21.*

The structure of the skin
The skin is made up of two layers, the epidermis and the dermis. The uppermost level of the epidermis is a tough protective layer of dead cells that rub off constantly as they are replaced by cells moving up from below. Under the dermis is a deep layer of subcutaneous fat.

Layer of subcutaneous fat

17

The epidermis

The epidermis is a multi-layered, self-renewing structure that varies in thickness from less than .004 inch on the eyelids to nearly .04 inch on the palms of the hands and soles of the feet.

GOING UP!

The epidermis renews itself constantly by cell division at its deepest layer, the basal layer. Keratinocyte cells produced by division in the basal layer are pushed toward the surface to become, in turn, the prickle cell layer, the granular layer, and—last of all—the horny layer, also called the stratum corneum, where they die. As the cells ascend toward the surface, they alter in structure and function. The time it takes for cells to pass from the basal cell layer to the horny layer is about 14 days. It takes another 14 days or so for cells in the horny layer to die and be rubbed off by daily wear and tear.

The epidermis varies in depth from 5 cells to 30 cells, depending on the part of the body. The thickness of the skin at any one part of the body always remains constant: The cells lost at the skin surface are balanced by new skin cells produced in the basal layer. Complex systems of cell growth regulation come into action to speed up or slow down cell division and maturation in the epidermis.

4 **The horny layer** (*stratum corneum*) *sits above the granular layer. By now the cells are flattened, with no nuclei or granules. The cells of the horny layer overlap each other like tiles, with the edges stuck together with a fatty "cement" ideal for waterproofing purposes. The horny layer varies in thickness according to the region of the body; it is thickest on the soles of the feet.*

3 **The granular layer** *is made up of flattened keratinocytes that contain not only granules of the protein keratohyalin but also lamellar granules that produce a "cement" that binds the cells together.*

2 **The prickle cell layer** *is composed mainly of keratinocytes packed closely together.*

1 **The basal layer cells** *are shaped like upturned bricks. They are anchored to a basement membrane from which threads extend down to anchor the membrane to the upper dermis.*

Melanocytes

Interspersed among the basal cells are the melanocytes, adapted nerve tissue cells that send out projections called dendrites between the epidermal cells. They produce the melanin that gives skin its color (see pages 28–29).

Merkel cells (or disks)

These cells are concentrated in areas around hair follicles in the basal layer, and probably transmit the sensation of light touch to the brain. Other nerve endings in the skin are sensitive to deeper pressure and temperature changes.

Inside view
*Here, the top covering of the
horny layer of the epidermis
has been peeled back, revealing
the pattern of the flattened
cells beneath.*

*Approximately
30,000 dead skin cells
are shed from the
epidermis every minute.*

KERATIN—WONDER SUBSTANCE

The epidermis is largely made up of
keratin—a protein that in effect provides the
body with a protective coating. It is keratin
that keeps too much moisture from
evaporating from the surface of the skin.
Keratin is virtually impenetrable by harmful
substances and also has antibacterial
properties. Keratin is also a major
constituent of the epidermal appendages,
the hair and nails.

Keratinocytes

Ninety-five percent of all cells in the epidermis are
keratinocytes—these are the cells that slowly move upward
from the basal layer to the skin's surface. They contain
keratin—the main structural protein of the epidermis.
Threads of keratin within keratinocytes in the basal and
prickle cell layers gradually combine to form bundles
that interweave and then become stuck together by a
"cement" produced by granules in the granular layer. By
the time they reach the horny layer, they form a mat that is an
almost impenetrable barrier that stops substances from passing
into and out of the body.

Langerhans cells

These are found in the prickle cell layer, and, like
melanocytes, they are dendritic cells. The first
line of defense against environmental hazards,
they seize harmful microorganisms and
deliver them to lymphocytes in the dermis so
an immune response can be generated.

The dermis

The dermis is the layer of connective tissue that lies between the epidermis above and the subcutaneous fat below. Its function is to support the epidermis structurally and nutritionally.

HOLDING IT ALL TOGETHER

The dermis is a network of interwoven fibers, composed principally of collagen and including a significant amount of elastin, which gives the skin its great strength and elasticity. These fibers are embedded in a strong ground substance of complex carbohydrates—mucopolysaccharides— that act as structural components in the connective tissue. Also within the dermis are several different types of cells—fibroblasts, mast cells, and macrophages—each with a different function. In addition, the dermis contains blood vessels, lymphatic vessels, nerves, and muscles. Nerve endings in the dermis act as receptors that pick up the sensations of light and heavy touch, pain, heat, and cold.

Merkel cell

Collagen *is the predominant fiber in the dermis. It is packed into bundles to give the skin strength and prevent tearing. Elastic fibers mingled with the collagen help the skin return to its original shape after movement or injury.*

Sweat gland

Macrophages *are a type of phagocyte. Their job is to consume cellular waste material and other debris, including bacteria.*

The thickness of the dermis varies from .12 inch or more on the soles of the feet to just .02 inch in the eyelids.

Fibroblasts *make up the majority of the cells in the dermis. They produce the connective tissue that "knits" the dermis together and tend to be located near collagen and elastin fibers.*

Subcutaneous fat layer

Blood vessels *in the skin help with temperature regulation. The network of vessels just above the subcutaneous fat also supplies the sweat glands and hair follicles.*

Basal layer of the epidermis

The ground substance *of the dermis is a semisolid gel in which fibers and cells are embedded. It holds water but allows nutrients, hormones and waste products to pass through. It lubricates the collagen and elastin fibers when the skin moves and also provides bulk, allowing the dermis to act as a shock absorber.*

A basement membrane *separates the epidermis and dermis.*

A Meissner's corpuscle *is a type of touch receptor.*

Mast cells *are specialized cells that spring into action when challenged by external injury or foreign substances. Granules inside each cell release histamine and other chemicals that play an important role in the inflammatory response to infection.*

Lymphocytes *are white blood cells involved in protecting the body from infection. They move between the lymphatic system and the bloodstream.*

Pacinian corpuscles *are one of several kinds of touch receptors found in the dermis—see pages 22–23.*

SUBCUTANEOUS FAT

The subcutaneous fat layer that sits below the dermis separates the skin from underlying bones and muscles. It is made up of loose connective tissue intermingled with fat cells. Its thickness varies depending on its location within the body. The boundary between the dermis and subcutaneous layer is generally indistinct; the one merges into the other.

Touch

The skin is packed with sensory receptors that give your body its sense of touch. This provides the brain with vital clues about the body in relation to its environment so it can act accordingly, such as withdrawing fingers from heat.

MAKING SENSE OF YOUR ENVIRONMENT

Sensory receptors within the epidermis and dermis can pick up touch, pain, heat, and cold. Sensory nerves vary in complexity, but all react to physical sensations, converting them into nerve impulses that are transmitted along the central nervous system to the thalamus inside the brain. In the thalamus, these impulses are identified and relayed to the appropriate sensory regions of the brain. Every second, billions of signals are transmitted to the brain from stimuli all over the body and are processed to create a sensory image and warn of any danger. The sensory receptor cells that lie within the epidermis or the upper dermis tend to be very sensitive to touch and heat; others located deeper within the dermis specialize in detecting heavier pressure.

Touch receptors

Touch receptors are types of sensory receptors. They range from free nerve endings to more complex tactile receptors enclosed in capsules of connective tissue. There are touch receptors all over the body, but some areas of skin—notably the palms, soles, and lips—have more than others and as a result are more sensitive to touch and pain.

Sensation and communication

Touching the skin has great psychological importance: Stroking and cuddling promotes emotional development, learning, and growth in newborn infants, and touching is known to enhance emotional well-being in people of all ages. Parts of the skin are also considered to be erogenous zones.

The skin has about a million nerve endings; most of these are in the skin on the face and hands, with relatively few on the back.

Epidermis

Blood vessels

Free nerve endings *are prevalent throughout the upper part of the dermis. They protrude into the epidermis.*

Dermis

Merkel's cells sense continuous light touch and pressure against the skin. Unlike other touch receptors, they are not covered by a capsule of connective tissue.

Meissner's corpuscles are especially sensitive touch receptors that are found in the upper dermis of the fingertips and palms, the lips, the soles of the feet, eyelids, nipples, and external genitalia.

Ruffini's corpuscles are touch receptors located deeper in the dermis; they pick up heavy prolonged touch and pressure.

Pacinian corpuscles detect the rapid movement (vibration) of tissues and changes in pressure; they are found deep in the dermis, close to muscles and joints, and in the wall of the bladder.

23

Protecting the body

The skin protects the body from the environment and from infection. Various mechanisms come into play to ensure that this protection is effective.

A BARRIER TO INFECTION

The skin's first line of defense is its robust, protective outer layer. Keratin, collagen, and elastin combine to form a tough but flexible covering. Sebum helps keep the skin supple. Pigment in skin protects against ultraviolet radiation by absorbing and scattering the rays and by scavenging free radicals. In addition, the dryness and constant shedding of dead skin cells, the benign microorganisms (mostly bacteria) that normally live on the skin, the fatty acids of sebum, and the lactic acid of sweat, all combine to repel invading bacteria, viruses, fungi, and parasites. Langerhans' cells in the epidermis and lymphoid tissue also play an active role in monitoring the skin for foreign substances and particles, acting quickly to eliminate them.

How invaders breach the skin

Despite these protective measures, infectious organisms can enter the skin in various ways. Natural openings abound: sweat pores, hair follicles, and sebaceous gland openings all allow bacteria, viruses, and fungal infections to enter. Broken skin or insect bites can be the port of entry for diseases such as malaria. Warm, moist areas are prone to fungal infections such as athlete's foot.

Hair shaft

Horny layer of the skin—the stratum corneum

Sebum on the skin

Sebum—an oily coating that cleans and seals

- *Sebaceous glands are located on the skin wherever there are hair follicles. They are larger and more numerous on the scalp, face, chest, and back. Most open into hair follicles; the only exceptions to these are sebaceous glands on the eyelids, in the genital area, and on the nipples.*
- *The sebum secreted by sebaceous glands is an oily compound containing various fatty substances. It enables the skin's outermost layer to retain water and controls water loss from the epidermis. The free fatty acids in sebum act as a disinfectant, helping to prevent bacteria and fungi from colonizing the skin.*
- *Sebum is produced at birth in response to maternal hormones, then disappears until puberty, when sebaceous glands develop, stimulated by androgens (the hormones produced by the testis), adrenal glands and—to a lesser extent—the ovaries.*

Sebum within a sebaceous gland

Dermis

Touch receptor

Hair follicle

Subcutaneous fat layer

A waterproof jacket

- *If you had no horny outer layer of the skin, you would lose significant amounts of water to the environment and would become dehydrated. The lipid bilayer, a fine layer of fats on the outer surface of the horny layer, keeps water from evaporating from the skin and makes it very difficult for water to enter from outside.*

- *There are times when the skin's ability to keep out water can become slightly impaired. This may happen when the horny layer is excessively dry or soggy, warmer than usual, or damaged in some way—perhaps by a detergent. Scientists take these factors into account when developing drug delivery systems or formulating cosmetic face creams.*

**Sweat expelled
onto the skin**

Epidermis

**Eccrine
sweat gland**

Blood vessel

White blood cells *move
toward a site of infection.*

The inflammatory response—localizing the damage

- *If foreign organisms do penetrate the body's protective defense barriers, the body's response is to generate inflammation of the immediate area to prevent infection from becoming more widespread.*

- *The damaged tissue releases chemicals that attract specialized scavenging cells—phagocyte-type white blood cells—to the infected area. Blood vessels inside the dermis dilate, increasing blood flow to the area. The walls of these tiny blood vessels become porous, allowing the phagocytes to move from the blood vessel into the area of tissue damage, where they engulf and destroy the invading microorganisms.*

- *The characteristic red, swollen, hot appearance of inflamed tissue is caused by the swollen blood vessels and the sharp increase in the number of cells in the tissue. The affected area becomes painful when the chemicals released during this process—such as serotonin and histamine—stimulate nerve endings in the dermis.*

Regulating temperature

Humans do not have a thick fur coat to provide warmth. Instead we rely on a complex system of specialized blood vessels in the skin and the action of the sweat glands to regulate heat loss and conservation.

WHEN THE BODY IS TOO HOT

When the temperature of the body increases and needs to be brought down again, the blood vessels near the surface of the skin dilate. This allows more blood to reach the skin so that heat is lost and the blood cools down. This brings a flushed appearance to the skin. How much the blood vessels dilate is controlled by nerves known as vasomotor fibers, which are controlled by the brain.

At the same time, eccrine sweat glands produce increased amounts of sweat, which evaporates on the surface of the skin to cool the skin. When the air is dry, the sweating mechanism is a very effective way of maintaining a tolerable body temperature. In humid heat, however, sweat cannot evaporate as easily, so the sweating mechanism is not so helpful, and the body may overheat.

WHEN THE BODY IS TOO COLD

If the body is too cold, the blood vessels close to the surface of the skin constrict to reduce the flow of blood. Warm blood is diverted into deeper blood vessels, and so heat is conserved (and the skin becomes paler).

The layer of subcutaneous fat under the dermis provides extra insulation and, in addition, the arrector pili muscles—the tiny muscles attached to hair follicles—contract, lifting the hairs until they become erect. This has the effect of pulling on the skin to produce goose bumps. In mammals with long, thick hair, the erect hairs trap a layer of warm air at the skin's surface; in humans this only has a small effect because human body hair is so short and fine. Fear and anger also make body hair stand on end.

Cooling down when too hot
The tiny blood vessels close to the skin's surface expand to increase the surface area of the blood vessel walls so that more heat can escape from the blood passing through.

Conserving heat when too cold
The tiny blood vessels near the skin's surface contract to reduce the amount of surface area from which heat can escape from the blood in the vessels.

There are about two-and-a-half million sweat glands on the surface of your skin.

A sweat gland is a long, coiled, hollow tube. Sweat is produced in the coiled part and then travels up the duct to where the gland emerges through a pore on the skin. The sweat is expelled and evaporates into the outside air. The gland shown here is an eccrine sweat gland—apocrine sweat glands open into a hair follicle.

Epidermis

Eccrine sweat glands are distributed through almost all of the body, with the greatest density being on the palms of the hands and the soles of the feet. These glands play a vital role in temperature regulation and are active from birth. Each gland has a coiled part deep in the dermis that secretes sweat and a duct that carries the sweat to the surface. The sweat consists of water, salts, and other waste products that need to be removed from the body. When the temperature outside the body is very hot, an eccrine duct can reabsorb salt to help the body conserve it.

Free nerve ending

Dermis

The duct connects the coiled part of the sweat gland to a pore on the skin's surface through which the sweat reaches the surface of the skin.

Apocrine sweat glands
These are mostly situated in the armpits and around the anus and genitals, with a few sometimes around the navel and nipples. They are larger than eccrine glands and become active at puberty, stimulated by production of the male sex hormone androgen. They have a secretory coil and a duct, much like eccrine glands, but the duct opens into a hair follicle, in the same way as a sebaceous gland. Their secretions include protein, carbohydrate, ammonia, and fats, and have nothing to do with temperature regulation. Apocrine gland sweat does not smell in itself, but a strong odor can result from the action of bacteria on the sweat. The glands that produce wax in the ear canal and the mammary glands of the breasts are specialized apocrine glands.

The coiled part in the dermis is where sweat first collects. The fluid that makes up sweat comes from the interstitial spaces between the cells. Fluid enters these spaces from the tiny blood vessels in the dermis.

Tiny blood vessels

The color of skin and hair

Compared with many creatures from the animal kingdom, humans have a rather limited color palette when it comes to skin and hair: We largely rely on shades of brown and red.

FROM BLACK TO WHITE

Brown skin—and hair—coloration is caused by melanin, with the intensity of color varying from almost white (no melanin) to almost jet black (a large amount). The amount of melanin our skin and hair contain is determined genetically.

MELANIN

Melanin is a pigment produced by specialized cells called melanocytes. These are found in the basal layer of the epidermis. Each melanocyte contains melanosomes, in which melanin is synthesized. These melanosomes are engulfed by keratinocyte cells, and it is differences in their behavior here that determine skin color.

There are also melanocytes in the bulbs of hair follicles (and in the retina of the eye). Melanocytes in a hair bulb are packaged into granules that pigment the hair shaft.

Hair color

Melanin produces a limited color palette in hair: shades of yellow, brown, red, and black.

Two forms of melanin color hair:

- *Eumelanin is the dark pigment that predominates in black and brunette hair. Pheomelanin is lighter and found in red and blonde hair. Many peoples' hair contains a mixture of the two: The more pheomelanin, the lighter the hair.*
- *The combination of pigments in any one head of hair is determined genetically. People of Celtic origin tend to have more pheomelanin than people of other races, hence the classic combination of red hair and very pale skin.*
- *The age at which hair starts to turn gray is also genetically determined. This occurs as production of the melanin that colors the hair slowly decreases and the cells in the medulla at the center of each terminal hair shaft become filled instead with tiny air bubbles that reflect light. Hairs without melanin appear to be white because of the way they reflect light.*

In pale-skinned people, *melanosomes are clustered together in melanosome complexes that gradually degenerate as the skin cells rise toward the surface.*

MELANIN AND SUN EXPOSURE

Melanin helps protect the skin from damage caused by ultraviolet (UV) radiation from the sun by absorbing the UV rays before they penetrate to deeper layers of the epidermis and dermis. UV rays are, however, useful for helping to produce vitamin D—important for calcium metabolism and strong, healthy bones—and so a moderate amount of UV radiation on the skin is beneficial, especially for people whose diet is viatmin D deficient.

Getting a suntan

Sunbathing leads to a suntan through two processes, one immediate and one taking place over the next few days. First, UV rays (mainly UVA) darken the skin by oxidising melanin that already exists; UVB stimulates the melanocytes to produce more melanin. The reason that some people tan more easily than others is because these people have more active melanocytes in their skin.

An evolutionary puzzle
Why do people have different colored skins that seem to be related to the part of the world from which they originate? The main reason is to protect them from sun damage: People in hotter countries have melanocytes in their skin that are more active and produce more melanin to absorb the potentially damaging UV rays from the sun. Also, it has been postulated that having a paler skin enables better UV absorption and therefore enhances vitamin D production for people living in regions of the world with less reliable sunshine.

Horny topmost layer of the epidermis

Granular layer of the epidermis

Melanosomes containing melanin *travel along the tentacle-like dendrites of each melanocyte. From here, they transfer to the keratinocytes that surround them.*

A melanocyte *with nucleus surrounded by cell membranes. Melanocytes are found in the basal cell layer of the epidermis, just above the dermis. They produce and store melanosomes.*

Keratinocyte

Prickle cell layer of the epidermis

In people born with darker skin *the melanosomes are greater in number and larger in size; they stay separate and remain active as they migrate upward, breaking down less rapidly than in people with paler skin.*

Basal layer of the epidermis

Basement membrane

Dermis

All about hair

Almost all of the surface of your skin is covered with hairs—be they obvious or not. The only hair-free zones are the palms of the hands, the soles of the feet, the nipples, the lips, and the eyelids.

HAIR TYPES

Hair is made of the protein keratin, which also makes up your nails and is a major constituent of the epidermis. There are two main types of hair:

- **Vellus hairs** are the short, fine, usually light-colored hairs that cover most of the body's surface. Vellus hairs on the body can change into terminal hairs in hirsutism, a condition of excessive hair growth.
- **Terminal hairs** are the longer, thicker, generally darker hairs that appear on the scalp, in the eyebrows and eyelashes, and in the armpits and genital area. Some groups of terminal hairs begin life as vellus hairs but change under the influence of hormones at puberty. These include the hair in the armpits and genital area, and some leg hair, and men also develop a beard and more body hair. If a man begins to lose the hair on his scalp, this reflects terminal hairs changing into vellus hairs.

WHAT IS HAIR FOR?

Most of the hair on your body performs no vital function—you could be hairless without any significant disturbance to your body's equilibrium. Some hair does, however, have a practical function: Eyelashes protect the eyes from foreign particles, eyebrows direct sweat away from the eyes, and hair on the scalp protects the head from ultraviolet radiation. Erect vellus hairs help conserve heat within the body when temperatures drop (see pages 26–27).

What makes hairs straight or curly?
In this colored electron micrograph of hair shafts protruding from a scalp, the roundness of each hair shaft indicates that these are straight hairs. The rounder the cross section of the shaft, the straighter the hair will be; the flatter the cross section, the more the hair will curl.

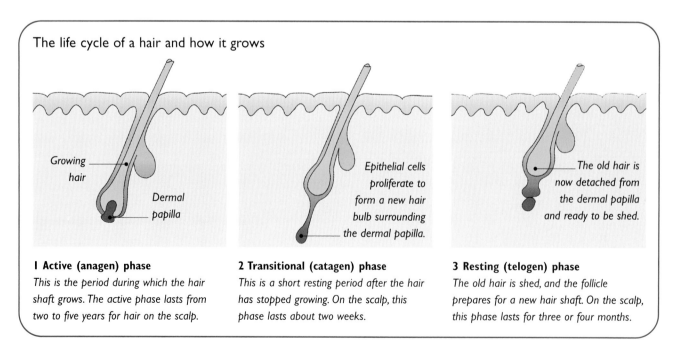

The life cycle of a hair and how it grows

Growing hair

Dermal papilla

Epithelial cells proliferate to form a new hair bulb surrounding the dermal papilla.

The old hair is now detached from the dermal papilla and ready to be shed.

1 Active (anagen) phase
This is the period during which the hair shaft grows. The active phase lasts from two to five years for hair on the scalp.

2 Transitional (catagen) phase
This is a short resting period after the hair has stopped growing. On the scalp, this phase lasts about two weeks.

3 Resting (telogen) phase
The old hair is shed, and the follicle prepares for a new hair shaft. On the scalp, this phase lasts for three or four months.

The cuticle *of a hair is made up of a thin layer of cells containing keratin. They overlap each other in a way similar to roof tiles, with the free margins pointing toward the tip of the hair. A "split end" may result if this layer wears away.*

The hair shaft *is the part of a hair that is visible above the surface of the skin.*

Epidermis

The cortex *consists of packed keratinocytes and contains the melanin pigment that gives the hair its color.*

The hair follicle *is under the skin's surface. It is a specialized tubular construction of epidermal cells that grows down into the dermis at an angle and contains the hair root.*

In the medulla, *at the center of a terminal hair, cells intermingle with air spaces. There is no medulla at all in vellus hairs.*

Basement membrane

Outer root sheath

There is a sebaceous gland *associated with each hair follicle. It helps lubricate the hair.*

Dermis

An arrector pili muscle *is attached to each hair follicle. When this bundle of muscle fibers contracts, the hair is pulled upright, creating a "goose bump."*

Sensory nerve endings

The hair bulb *at the lower end of the follicle encloses the dermal papilla. Included within the hair bulb are melanocytes and keratinocytes, which give the hair its color and texture.*

The dermal papilla *contains dividing cells and receives blood vessels and nerve endings that nourish the growing hair. It is from the dermal papilla that a new hair grows once the old hair has died.*

The ends of the line

As our principal instruments of touch, the fingertips are in constant use and, along with the vulnerable toes, are in need of extra protection. This is provided by the nails, which are also useful tools in themselves.

The skin on the fingertips is particularly well supplied with nerve endings. Each fingertip has more than 3000 touch receptors.

THE NAILS

The nail is, in fact, the evolutionary remnant of a mammalian claw. It consists of a plate of hardened and densely packed keratin. In addition to protecting the finger ends, the nails have valuable prying and picking skills.

How fast do nails grow?

The rate at which nails grow varies from person to person. Fingernails grow continuously and average between .02 and .05 inch per week. Toenails grow about a third more slowly. Nails grow faster when you are younger and faster in summertime than in winter, possibly because blood circulates at a faster rate in summer, triggering more rapid cell division. It takes about six months for a fingernail to grow from the matrix to the free edge and up to 18 months for the nail on the big toe to do the same. The nails on your dominant hand grow a little faster than those on your nondominant hand. Diseases of the nail, skin, or body can affect the growth rate of the nails generally. Nails do not continue to grow for a short time after death, as is sometimes thought, but the nail folds do shrink away from the nail plate, creating the illusion that the nail has grown.

The lateral nail fold *is the bulge of skin on either side of the nail, at the boundary of the epidermis and the nail.*

The nail plate *is a hard transparent form of keratin that grows outward from the nail matrix.*

The free edge *is the part of the nail that extends beyond the nail bed.*

The bone *at the fingertip is known as the terminal or distal phalanx.*

Epidermis

Dermis

The lunula *is the only part of the matrix that you can see. It looks like a pale "half-moon" at the base of the nail plate (lunula is Latin for "crescent-shaped moon").*

The cuticle *is an extension of the horny layer of the skin of the nail fold. It acts as a seal to protect the matrix from infection.*

Proximal nail fold

The nail bed *lies immediately beneath the nail plate.*

A layer of fat *surrounds the bone at the end of the finger.*

The matrix or root of the nail *runs from the proximal nail fold to the outer edge of the lunula. From this root, the nail plate grows over the nail bed, ending in a free edge at the fingertip. It is in the matrix that keratin is produced by cell division. Therefore, if the matrix is destroyed, the nail can't grow back.*

WHAT IS A FINGERPRINT?

On the fingertips, the outermost layer of skin forms tiny ridges that make up the distinctive patterns that we call our fingerprints. These ridges are found all over the palms of the hands and the soles of the feet. The patterns they form are unique to you (only identical twins share the same patterns). The ridges follow the same patterns that are created below the skin's surface, where the dermis and epidermis join by means of interlocking projections down from the epidermis (called rete ridges) and up from the dermis (dermal papillae). The projections lock the dermis and epidermis together.

Loop

Arch

Whorl

Distinctive patterns
Loops are the most common fingertip ridge patterns; arches are the least common. Everyone has a unique pattern of loops, whorls, and arches.

A lifetime of skin, hair, and nails

From birth through adolescence to middle age and beyond, your skin and hair slowly change in appearance. These changes are mostly caused by the natural maturing and aging processes, but the effects of too much sun exposure can also become apparent as the years go by.

SMOOTH AS SILK?

A baby's skin is often hailed as being perfect, but this may be far from the case for newborns. In general, a baby's skin is thinner, less oily, and more fragile than that of an adult, so it becomes irritated, sore, and sunburned more easily. Prominent sebaceous glands or whitish bumps may appear; both should disappear naturally in a few weeks. Babies don't sweat as efficiently as adults, and sometimes little blisters caused by blocked sweat ducts can develop.

A baby's hair is usually very fine, and babies are frequently born blond and develop darker hair as they become older. A premature baby may be born with fine, long hairs—called lanugo hairs—covering the head, shoulders and back. These form in the fetus at around 20 weeks, but they are normally shed before a full-term birth.

Babies are born with soft, rapidly growing nails that are almost always perfect—congenital abnormalities of the nails are very rare.

TEENAGE TRAUMA

Both sexes begin to produce the hormone testosterone, which causes the sebaceous glands in hair follicles and pores to produce the natural oil known as sebum. When the body overproduces sebum, dead skin cells tend to clog the sebaceous glands, creating the blemishes that characterize acne. Sebaceous gland activity can also make hair greasier. Hormones also trigger the conversion of vellus hairs in the genital areas and armpits into terminal hairs—as well as the growth of facial hair and more terminal body hair in adolescent boys.

THE MIDDLE YEARS

In the middle years, the dermis begins to hold less water and fat so skin loses its "roundness" and starts to sag. The skin becomes less resilient because fewer elastic fibers are produced. It becomes dryer in response to less sebum production, and cell renewal takes longer, so older cells remain on the skin surface longer, causing creases and wrinkles. This process is apparent in most people by their late 40s; in those who have spent time in the sun or who smoke, it becomes apparent earlier.

Hair begins to turn gray, and some people start to lose their hair. The age at which this happens is genetically determined, but, like the skin, hair is also affected by UV radiation from the sun, becoming dry and coarse after a lot of sun exposure.

As the body gets older, the nails, particularly the toenails, harden, and life starts to take its toll on the feet and nails, with the development of problems such as hard skin.

SIGNS OF LIFE

As the body ages, the skin becomes increasingly thinner and more wrinkled because of loss of elasticity, collagen, moisture, and fat. Exposure to UV rays speeds up this aging process, especially in Caucasian skin. In addition, the number of melanocytes (which contain the pigment melanin) in the skin gradually decrease with advancing age, making skin even more susceptible to UV damage and so also to skin cancer.

With advancing years, the amount of sebum produced falls (slightly in men, significantly in women) so that skin becomes drier and less supple. The amount of collagen in the skin decreases by about 1 percent per year through adult life—more in women after menopause—causing skin to sag. Fewer fibroblasts are present in the dermis, meaning that wounds heal more slowly. Over the age of 70, the skin is less able to regulate body heat, which is why the elderly are so much more susceptible to the effects of severe cold weather.

A day in the life of the skin and hair

It's the weekend, and you have the opportunity to spend time with family and friends and to take things at a more leisurely pace than normal. Your skin and hair, however, cannot take a break from their work of protecting you from the outside world.

SKIN CONSCIOUS

Your skin is constantly working to keep you healthy. It helps cool you when you are hot and warm you when you are cold; it works hard to keep out—and limit the damage caused by—ultraviolet radiation and invading microorganisms. You may not be conscious of it for much of the day, but your skin is vital to your well-being.

8:00 A.M. Rise and shine

You wake up feeling too hot. In response, the tiny blood vessels close to the surface of your skin have dilated in order to lower your internal temperature. As you head for the shower, nerve endings in your soles sense pressure and the coolness of the wooden floor. You end your shower with a quick blast of cold water, and the little blood vessels in your skin constrict to prevent you from becoming too cold. You apply underarm antiperspirant deodorant: The antiperspirant temporarily stops the production of sweat, and the deodorant ensures that any sweat is odorless by inhibiting the action of bacteria on the skin.

10:30 A.M. Saturday morning shopping

After dropping the children off at their friends' house, you head for the mall. You noticed this morning that your shampoo and conditioner are running low and that the skin on your face seems drier than normal. The pharmacist recommends a change in your normal moisturizer. You are also concerned that you have picked up a wart on one of your regular swimming sessions and ask the pharmacist to recommend an over-the-counter medication to deal with it.

1:00 P.M. Out of the afternoon sun

You have a date for lunch with a friend—a regular weekend treat. But the sun is high and the day is warm, so you choose a sidewalk table under the awning: Ultraviolet intensity is at its greatest when the sun is overhead, so you take care to stay out of the sun as much as possible between 11 A.M. and 3 P.M. At the very least, ultraviolet radiation hastens the development of wrinkles, which appear when the dermis loses its elastic recoil so that it doesn't snap back into shape properly. When skin is exposed to ultraviolet radiation for long periods of time on a regular basis, the elastic fibers within the dermis clump together and lose their shape.

3:00 P.M. Park and ride

It's a beautiful afternoon, so instead of going straight home when you pick up the kids, you all go to the park. First you make sure everyone has sunblock on any exposed skin, and you slap on hats, too. Although the peak sun hours have passed, it's still hot, and after the kids have run around for half an hour, you are worried that they might be overheating. Children get hot faster than adults and produce more internal heat, but their real problem is the immaturity of their sweating ability: They can't sweat enough to dissipate excess heat by evaporation. You all sit in the shade of a tree and drink a rehydrating bottle of juice.

8:00 P.M. Food for friends

Back at home, you bathe the children, taking care to dry them well, and put them to bed. Then it's time to relax with friends over supper. For starters, you have a small serving of chicken liver paté, rich in vitamin A, a vital nutrient in preserving healthy skin. You follow this with tuna salad—its essential fatty acids are good for your skin. A glass of wine brings a flush to your cheeks, so you alternate with plain water, which will keep your skin and you hydrated.

2

Keeping your skin, hair, and nails healthy

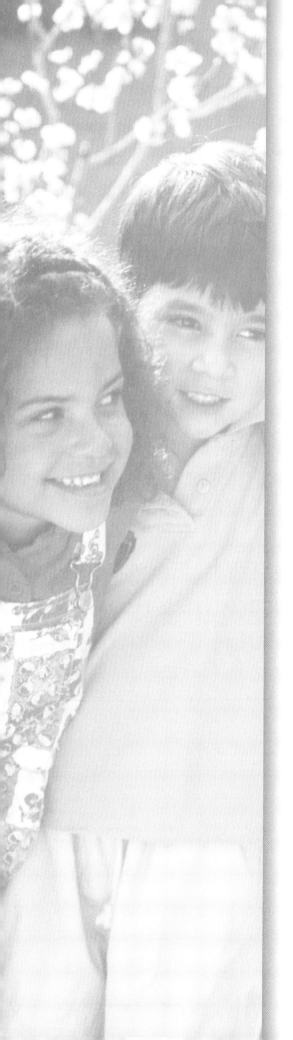

TAKE CHARGE OF YOUR SKIN HEALTH

No part of your body tells your life story better than your skin. Changes as you age, as well as many ongoing factors—work, the environment, diet, whether you smoke or drink alcohol—all affect what your skin looks and feels like. The appearance of your skin also reflects your general health.

41 *As we get older, our skin and hair change. By responding to these changes, we can keep our skin and hair in optimum condition.*

46 *Understanding the potential damage the environment can do to skin and hair enables us to take preventative measures.*

51 *Some medications can cause skin reactions. If you are starting treatment, look out for skin changes; most reactions soon disappear.*

52 *Simple daily care routines can make a big difference to your skin and hair. It is not essential to use large amounts of products.*

61 *Body hair removal can irritate the skin. Read about the methods available and recommended for different skin types and areas of the body.*

63 *Regular nail maintenance can help reduce the effects of environmental damage and physical stress on your nails.*

The changing face of skin and hair

Our skin and hair change as we age, because of the hormonal changes we go through and the environmental factors we are exposed to. Most of us will suffer some kind of problem with our skin and hair at some time in our lives.

HOW SKIN CHANGES WITH AGE

Some changes to the skin are intrinsic to the aging process of the tissue itself, some are caused by influences such as hormones and disease processes, and some result from environmental factors. In areas of the skin exposed to the environment, 90 percent of the signs of aging are caused by environmental factors, mainly UV radiation from the sun.

Babies

The surface area of the skin of a newborn baby is much larger in proportion to the volume of the body, so babies are more vulnerable to heat and fluid loss than older children and adults are. The skin's barrier system is not fully activated, so babies lose extra water even though their sweat glands are not yet activated.

During the first few weeks of life the mother's hormones are circulating and stimulate the baby's sebaceous glands. Babies also have a blood vessel system that is much more reactive, so a baby's skin color may change from pink to bright red within a few minutes. Don't overdress a baby: In hot weather a shirt diaper may be all that are needed, but watch for signs of cooling—babies cool down as fast as they overheat.

These factors mean that drugs applied to a baby's skin can be absorbed much more quickly and in larger amounts, leading to potential toxicity problems. Babies' skin is more vulnerable to chemical, physical, and microbial attack because their defense systems have not matured completely.

They are prone to diaper rash, in which the skin is irritated by prolonged contact with the chemicals in urine. To prevent this,
• use an effective barrier cream;
• change soiled diapers promptly;
• allow babies diaper-free time to get air to their skin.

Young children

Genetic predisposition, influenced by the environment, contributes to the development of several of the most common skin diseases of childhood, such as atopic eczema. In families with a tendency to atopic problems (such as eczema, asthma, and hay fever) we do not know precisely what sparks off the conditions in each individual, but these conditions are becoming much more common. Atopic eczema may be provoked by allergens such as dust mites or cow's milk in the diet. It was thought that avoiding cow's milk and breastfeeding a baby might reduce that risk, but recent evidence may disprove this.

Less is more
When cleansing infants' skin, use specially formulated products that are fragrance-free and have as few ingredients as possible.

At school

As a child grows and starts nursery school, contact with infectious diseases such as chicken pox increases. A child with chicken pox may not feel very ill, but the spots are itchy and it's very difficult for a child not to scratch. For a young child, cotton gloves may be the answer, but for an older child a cooling lotion such as calamine or aloe vera, a cool bath, or an oatmeal bath can help to ease the itching.

Many activities put the skin in contact with potential irritant chemicals, and contact dermatitis can appear. Nickel allergy and rubber footwear sensitivity are examples of this type of problem. Trauma to the skin in the form of scrapes, cuts, and bruises become an everyday event, but these should not be a problem if cuts are kept clean and treated with antiseptic cream.

Puberty

During puberty most teenagers suffer from blemishes or acne of some sort (see below). Keep your skin clean by washing gently twice a day with a mild soap. Avoid squeezing spots—this can introduce infection. Instead, apply a topical salicylic product to the area using a cotton swab, to gently dry blemishes.

When girls gain fat during puberty, the skin on the buttocks and thighs can develop a dimpled appearance. This is known as cellulite and is completely normal for women. Although losing weight can make the dimples appear less prominent, no amount of massaging or scrubbing techniques will make any difference.

The 20s

During your 20s, your skin starts to settle down after the upheaval of the teenage years, although oil (sebum) production may still be relatively high. Visible signs of aging can start to appear toward the end of your 20s as the regenerative processes begin to slow. Skin may show a shift toward dryness, and some people may notice the first lines forming around their eyes.

During your 20s a number of lifestyle choices can help slow the effects of aging. The most important is to reduce sun damage: Limit the time spent in the sun, wear sunscreen, and keep your body well-hydrated by drinking at least 2.5 quarts of water a day. If you smoke, try to stop: Smoking prematurely ages the skin. This is also a good time to start a skin-care routine, with daily cleansing and light moisturizing.

30-something

During your 30s, you will begin to see the first real signs of aging as collagen and elastin fibers decrease.

Fine, dry lines appear around the eyes, where the skin is at its thinnest. Increased water loss leads to drying, and this decreases the skin's natural protective barrier. Broken veins show up as tiny red dots and "laugh lines" will run deeper on the side you sleep on. Lifestyle changes are less dramatic, but stress can be a critical issue. The regular late nights you enjoyed in your 20s now bring puffy dark circles under your eyes.

Both men and women should wear a sunscreen of at least SPF 15, and moisturizer can be used daily. Eye creams and gels can also become useful at this stage.

The middle years

If you have taken reasonably good care of your skin, avoided excess sun, and are healthy, the signs of aging should be minor for both men and women. However, deeper lines form around the mouth and eyes, furrows appear on the forehead, and age spots may develop. After age 45, a thinning of the skin begins. The skin looks less plump and smooth and loses its youthful glow because of fewer blood vessels in the skin.

At this age all skin-care products used should be hydrating. A rich moisturizer can help to reinvigorate tired, slack skin and improve texture.

60 plus

The changes in skin tone experienced in the 50s continue throughout the 60s and beyond. The skin gets drier and looser as less oil is produced and as a result becomes more wrinkled. The skin lightens in color because of decreased circulation, and wound healing is slower. Most people over 60 find that moisturizer is the best form of skin care.

10–20 YEARS

Teenagers and acne, blemishes, and blackheads

Acne is one of the most common skin disorders. It is characterized by blackheads, whiteheads, and pimples, especially on the face, back, and chest. Acne is mainly seen in adolescents and tends to be slightly more severe in males.

Most acne is caused by an overproduction of sebum by the sebaceous glands in the skin. This is triggered by increased levels of androgen (male) hormones in both males and females during puberty.

Excess sebum can cause the follicle openings on the skin to become blocked. The sebum can harden and darken, forming blackheads. If the follicles are sealed by keratin (dead skin cells) the sebum hardens under the skin to form whiteheads. In both cases, bacteria can multiply in the sebum, causing inflammation. This attracts white blood cells that form pus; if pustules develop deep into the skin, painful nodules form.

Acne products can help by killing the bacteria that cause inflammation; if these do not work, a doctor may prescribe medication (see page 113). Because acne can affect the way people feel about themselves, it is worth seeking professional help.

PREGNANCY

The hormonal changes in pregnancy can lead to a number of changes to the skin, hair, and nails. Most of these are advantageous for women, although there can be downsides.

Some of the skin changes are related to the increase in blood supply to the skin. This can result in the characteristic "glow" of pregnancy, when many women say their skin feels healthier. Many women get fewer blemishes because hormonal changes can reduce sebum production. Eating better and avoiding smoking and alcohol may also have benefits for the skin.

Skin diseases such as eczema and psoriasis may improve during pregnancy, but they can become worse. Some women find that red palms and small spider-like blood vessels can develop.

Pregnancy also brings an increase in skin pigmentation, particularly in brunettes. Areas of the skin that are already dark—such as the nipples, areolae, genital area, and the midline of the abdominal wall—can become darker. Up to 70 percent of women develop a condition called melasma (also called chloasma), in which the skin color of the forehead, temples, and central part of the face darkens. These changes are caused by the increase in estrogen in the bloodstream and usually settle down when the pregnancy ends, though some women are left with permanent changes. Mole size and activity may also increase.

Nails grow faster and can become brittle and raised from the nail bed. Massaging petroleum jelly into the cuticles may help.

Keeping the skin supple
Some women develop stretch marks that fade after the pregnancy but do not entirely disappear. Many women claim that certain creams and lotions are effective if massaged into the skin during pregnancy, but generally whether a woman develops stretchmarks is a matter of luck: There is no really effective treatment.

Changes to hair texture
Many women find that their hair becomes thicker during pregnancy. This is because estrogen keeps a larger proportion of hairs in the actively growing phase. Oil production increases, so hair that was dry before pregnancy may become shiny; hair that was oily, however, may appear lank.

Freckles are more common in children and in people with pale skin and fair or red hair. They may fade almost completely in the winter and darken again in the sun.

Some freckles persist even in the absence of the sun; these are called lentigos, or liver spots (page 148). Despite the name, these are not linked to liver function. They tend to appear on sun-exposed sites. Liver spots usually appear during middle age. No treatment is needed but they can, rarely, be associated with the development of melanoma.

HAIR GROWTH
The rate of hair growth varies around the body. Human vellus hair grows 0.0012 inch in 24 hours on the male forehead, 0.008 inch every 24 hours on the female thigh, 0.015 inch in 24 hours on the chin of a young male, and 0.02 inch per 24 hours on the crown of the scalp. Scalp hair grows faster in women than men but faster in boys than girls before puberty. Hair may grow faster depending on age, genetics, and hormonal state. Growth of body hair peaks between the ages of 50 and 69.

Straight or curly?
Whether a hair is straight or curly depends on the shape of the hair shaft. Straight hair has a circular cross section, curly hair has a flattened elliptical cross section, and wavy hair has a shape somewhere between a circle and a flattened ellipse. These factors vary according to racial origin.

Thinning and balding hair
As many adults age, their hair can become thinner and they experience some hair loss (see pages 85–87).

The freckle gene
Freckles are inherited, and as a person ages her freckles tend to become less noticeable. Apart from sun protection, no treatment is necessary.

NORMAL FRECKLES AND MOLES
Freckles and moles are very common and are usually harmless pigmented spots on the skin. Birthmarks are pigmented areas of skin varying in size and color (see page 136). The major problem for medical and lay people is deciding whether a mole may be a form of skin cancer: 30 percent of malignant melanomas—the least common but potentially fatal form of skin cancer—arise in a preexisting mole.

What is a mole?
Moles are collections of pigment-forming cells (melanocytes) situated in the epidermis or dermis. They can be present from birth (congenital) or develop afterward (acquired). The majority appear after birth but before age 20. They continue to develop and change until about the age of 40. Initially, the cells are at the basal layer of the epidermis but gradually sink into the dermis, after which they grow and become raised.

It is important to check for any changes to moles that may suggest malignancy, including border and color irregularity and asymmetry.

Anyone who has more than about 50 moles or who has a family history of malignant melanoma or atypical moles should have them checked regularly by a doctor.

What are freckles?
Freckles, also called ephelides, are pale brown flat spots of concentrated pigment. They are usually less than a tenth of an inch in diameter with an irregular edge: Those that seem larger may be joined to another.

HAIR COLOR

Hair color is genetically controlled. Human hair color is under the control of at least four different genes. Dark hair predominates in the world, and ethnic differences among hair colors are very evident.

Hair pigmentation depends entirely on the presence of melanin, a pigment produced by melanocyte cells in the hair follicle, but the color we perceive also depends on the hair's physical condition. The range of colors produced by melanin is limited to shades of yellow, brown, red, and black.

Hair color often darkens with age, so a redheaded child may darken to brown or auburn in adulthood.

Hair color may also change because of nutritional deficiencies, particularly copper and protein deficiency. Hair also binds to inorganic elements such as copper, and a chlorinated swimming pool can turn blond hair green. Cobalt workers can develop blue hair, and indigo handlers can have deep blue hair. People who work with TNT sometimes develop reddish-brown hair.

The graying of hair

Graying hair is part of the aging process and is caused by a progressive reduction in melanocyte function. This results in a gradual dilution of pigment along individual hairs from normal to white and from one hair to another: This process is called canities. When there are few, if any, remaining melanocytes in the hair follicle, the hair appears white. The white color seen in the absence of melanin is caused by the reflection and refraction of light on the hair; there really is no color at all.

> **By the age of 50 at least half the population have at least 50 percent gray hair. In men, the beard and mustache go gray before the hair on the head.**

Close examination of graying hair frequently reveals a small precentage of white hairs among a higher percentage of normal dark pigmented hairs.

The age at which the graying process starts is genetically determined: On average it begins between the mid-30s and mid-40s. Premature graying has been defined as onset before 20 in Caucasians and 30 in negroid people. It is thought to have a genetic base and is commonly associated with autoimmune disorders such as pernicious anemia and thyroid disease. Some people have localized patches of white hairs caused by the absence of melanocytes or a deficiency in follicle function.

Can hair really turn white overnight?

Hair can't turn white overnight because hair is dead and the only way to change its color is with dye. However, a condition known as diffuse alopecia areata may occur in someone with a mix of white and pigmented hairs (or "salt and pepper" hair). This condition—caused by enormous stress or emotional upheaval—results in sudden, substantial hair loss. For unknown reasons it seems to affect mostly pigmented hairs, leaving white hairs untouched, so it appears that the person's hair has become white "overnight." After an episode of alopecia areata, new hairs often grow in white but become pigmented.

IT'S NOT TRUE!

"Shaving makes your hair grow faster/curly/thicker"

Shaving will not make your hair grow thicker, faster, or curlier. Hair is dead protein, so cutting it won't make any difference to how it grows.

Hair may initially feel coarser after shaving, but this is caused by the feel of blunt hair ends after being cut with a razor. If shaving actually increased hair growth, it would essentially be a cure for male pattern baldness and many more men would have shaved heads in the short term.

Avoiding risks to the skin and hair

Our appearance determines to a large extent how we think of ourselves, and self-image and self-esteem are vitally bound up with our looks. This makes an awareness of the factors that might harm how we look important.

A major function of the skin is to prevent the environment from damaging the body's vulnerable tissues. All parts of the skin contribute to this protective role. The skin can react in several different ways to internal illnesses and to the world around us.

Many people take their skin for granted, but it has several basic needs. First, it needs to be kept clean. Second, it needs to be protected from sunlight and the environment. It shows its reaction to environmental factors in several different ways, including eczema, blistering, acne, rashes, and discoloration.

Skin comes into contact with a variety of chemical substances, some of which are fairly harmless and others that are dangerous. And although toxic substances are capable of injuring all who come into contact with them, some individuals have more sensitive skin than others.

In general, people with darker skins are at less risk from irritant damage and UV damage—fair-skinned and red-haired individuals suffer much more. The reason for these differences is not known, but people with fair skin have high UV sensitivity and are at an increased risk of developing skin problems caused by chemical irritants.

Even everyday things in places we would regard as natural and harmless can unexpectedly cause a severe problem.

HOUSEHOLD IRRITANTS

Most everyday substances such as dish soap, bleach, oven cleaner, and detergents are fairly harmless with occasional contact, but repeated exposure can damage the skin. These substances can penetrate and irritate the epidermis, causing dermatitis. Repeated irritation leads to so-called chemical irritant eczema. This is an inflammatory response by the skin to the injury. Toxic chemicals such as acids can remove the surface layer of the skin by destroying the cells, leaving a weeping bare area or skin ulcer.

In addition to causing eczema, chemicals may cause blistering or abnormalities in pigmentation. Depigmentation can be caused by materials that damage the pigment-producing cells, such as some rubber additives.

People with sensitive skin find that some cosmetic products cause irritant or allergic reactions. The products most likely to cause a problem are eye and facial cosmetics, deodorants, hair dyes, and soaps. If a reaction occurs, cosmetics should not be used and, if necessary, topical steroid cream can be prescribed until the reaction subsides.

DOMESTIC IRRITATIONS

At home or in the garden the skin can be exposed to many irritant substances. Regular exposure can damage the skin's protective barriers, so it is always best to take preventative measures.

COVER UP
When gardening, wear protective gloves to protect your skin from scratches and contact with any chemicals.

BE KIND TO YOUR HANDS
Applying moisturizer will help rehydrate the skin, and it can also provide an effective barrier to prevent further moisture loss.

BE LAUNDRY WISE
If you have sensitive skin, use fragrance- and dye-free detergent and double rinse your clothes to remove residue.

What you can do

- Avoid prolonged exposure to potential irritants: Wear gloves when handling chemicals.
- Wash and dry hands thoroughly and use a moisturizer; massage it into the nails and cuticles too.
- If you have sensitive skin, use hypoallergenic products (page 54).

GARDEN HAZARDS

Our lives are inextricably bound up with plants, whether we are growing them, cooking and eating them, or arranging them for display. Some occupations bring people into daily contact with potentially hazardous plants and woods. People at risk for occupational skin problems include gardeners, nursery workers, fruit pickers, florists, flower arrangers, grocers, farmers, foresters, and botanists.

Some plants are known to cause skin rashes, and it may be that they have survived better for being dangerous to pick or eat. More commonly, however, the reaction may be caused by a chemical the plant produces. Plants that are known to cause irritant eczema include primroses, ivy, euphorbia, daffodil bulbs, and dieffenbachia, a common office plant. Other plants only cause problems when we are also in the sun. Such phototoxic reactions are caused by a relatively small number of species, including

- **Umbellifers** Vegetables such as celery, carrots, and parsnips; herbs such as dill, cumin, and parsley; ornamental plants; and weeds such as cow parsley and giant hogweed.
- **Rutaceae** These include citrus fruits, rue, and burning bush.
- **Figs**

The chemical involved in all these reactions is psoralens, a natural fungicide produced by plants. This interacts with the DNA of mammalian cells, and when UV rays fall on the area it can produce an acute inflamed blistered area of skin. The skin rash urticaria can be produced by some plants, such as the stinging nettle, injecting the irritant into the skin; the rash appears at the point of contact. In other cases, eating the plant can provoke urticaria all over the body. Foods such as green peppers, strawberries, onions, and tomatoes may cause such reactions.

Skin reactions when gardening can also be caused by such irritants as rubber in gloves or the stinging hairs of the brown-tail moth, which lives in garden sheds.

Weedkillers and insecticides can damage the nails. This can vary from causing a white band across the nail to total loss of the nail.

What you can do

- Wear non-latex gloves when you are gardening.
- Avoid foods that cause a rash.
- Avoid the sun when gardening: Choose cool times of day.
- Use organic weedkillers and check the safety of any insecticides used.
- Don't grow plants that cause skin irritation: If they are already in your garden, have them removed.

CHOOSE SHOES WITH CARE
To keep the skin on your feet healthy, buy shoes made from breathable materials such as leather or canvas.

TAKE TIME OUT
Massage is a soothing form of relaxation, and the firm but gentle hand movements increase oxygen and blood flow to the skin.

OIL CLEANUP
Lubricating oils used by mechanics can cause acne and dermatitis, so clean your skin thoroughly.

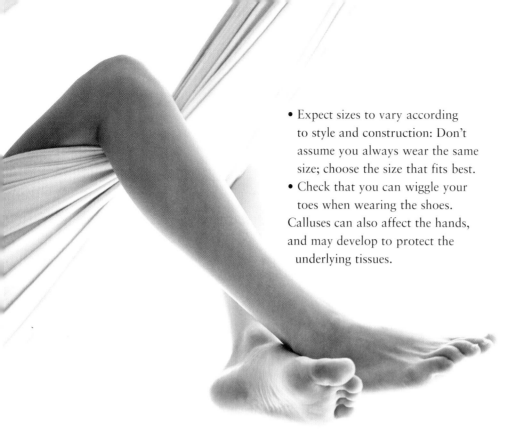

- Expect sizes to vary according to style and construction: Don't assume you always wear the same size; choose the size that fits best.
- Check that you can wiggle your toes when wearing the shoes. Calluses can also affect the hands, and may develop to protect the underlying tissues.

Forgotten feet

If you spend all day on your feet, fill a large bowl with warm water and add some bubble bath for a soothing and relaxing foot spa.

SHOES AND THE SKIN

Many minor but painful foot problems such as calluses and corns are caused by poorly fitting shoes. These small pads of hard skin develop at sites under pressure. People who spend their time walking barefoot are prone to developing large areas of thickened skin on the soles of the feet. These develop as a way for the foot to protect itself from injury, but they can become cracked, painful, and infected.

When buying shoes:

- Choose leather or canvas: Both materials breathe and mold to your feet.
- Always have your feet measured: Feet can spread with age, so your shoe size may alter over the years.
- Shop for shoes at the end of the day, when your feet will have swollen to their maximum extent.

STRESS AND THE SKIN

It is generally believed that stress can cause illness, and this applies to skin conditions, too. Stress can exacerbate several preexisting skin conditions such as acne, psoriasis, and rosacea. It is also believed that outbreaks of these conditions can be triggered by a single stressful event.

There is also a self-induced skin disease, dermatitis artefacta, which may be related to psychological problems. Picking, scratching, and rubbing the skin; pulling out hair; and damaging nails by picking can all lead to serious skin problems.

One of the best things you can do for the health of your body, which will also have a positive impact on your skin, is to find out what stresses you and to take steps to relieve it.

Relief strategies

- Take a break.
- Buy a self-help book or video.
- Learn to meditate or do yoga.
- Eat well and avoid alcohol.
- Get enough sleep.

YOUR OCCUPATION AND YOUR SKIN

An occupational skin disease (OSD) is any skin disorder caused by a person's work. An existing skin disorder may also be made worse by work activities, and such cases are also considered to be OSDs. Skin diseases are one of the most common forms of work-induced illness, so it is important to know whether you are at risk from the type of work that you do.

Skin reactions account for 40 percent of all occupational diseases.

Examples of occupational skin problems include

- contact dermatitis;
- irritant and allergic dermatitis; and
- worsening of preexisting skin diseases such as eczema.

Some skin cancers are also related to occupations. It is estimated that six million working days are lost ever year in the United States because of skin conditions.

People with the highest risk include hairdressers, printers, nurses, foundry workers, beauticians, machine tool operators, chemical and biological scientists, electroplaters, and vehicle assemblers. Anyone who has a history of eczema as a child might be advised to think carefully before pursuing one of these occupations.

Nails can also be damaged in occupations such as hairdressing, while artificial nail appliers have been known to develop sensitivity to the adhesive.

OBESITY

The skin is affected by obesity. Conditions such as intertrigo— skin infections of the groin, under the breasts, in the armpits—are common because microorganisms can flourish in the warm, moist areas created by folds of fat.

People who are seriously overweight can develop stretch marks on their abdomen and thighs that resemble those that occur in pregnancy. They are particularly common in adolescents who gain weight quickly and usually become less obvious after weight is lost.

People with severe obesity may develop insulin resistance, thought to be the precursor to type II diabetes. Various skin problems are associated with this, including a thickening and darkening of skin creases.

Irritating work
Hairdressers come into contact with a wide range of chemicals that can damage the surface layer of the skin and cause eczema.

SMOKING

Collagen fibers form the structural support in the dermis of the skin and are constantly being renewed. Smoking impedes this process, leading to premature aging of the skin. Smoking also reduces the blood supply to the skin by damaging the frail membrane lining the arteries. This can lead to loss of hair on the legs, shiny fragile skin, and delayed healing. The toenails can thicken and become deformed, and fingernails can split. The arch of the foot may also distort, leading to ulcers on the toes. This is many times worse in someone who already has diabetes.

A yellowish hair color is not uncommon in white or gray-haired heavy smokers because of the tar in cigarette smoke. The fingernails and fingers can be heavily discolored yellow and brown, stained by the tar.

The best advice for your skin is not to smoke, or if you do, to use every available resource to stop.

ALCOHOL

Alcohol has the reputation of giving people a red face. In fact, alcohol, hot drinks, spicy foods, emotion, UV light, and extremes of temperature can all precipitate flushing in a vulnerable individual. The blood vessels of the skin dilate, bringing extra blood to the skin surface, so the skin reddens and feels warm. For most people, alcohol-related flushing is only temporary and fades after a few hours.

In some people, the small blood vessels become fixed in dilation, so they appear red-faced and have tiny broken blood vessels on the skin of their face all the time. Alcohol may also raise the body's temperature, causing sweating.

Heavy drinking can lead to a dry, dull complexion. This is caused by the dehydrating effects of alcohol and is more noticeable in women. Minor skin infections are also more common because alcohol weakens the body's natural defense system. Alcohol poisoning is indicated by cold, clammy, pale, or bluish skin.

It is important to drink only in moderation (no more than two drinks a day for a woman and three for a man, and always have one or two alcohol-free days each week).

STREET DRUGS

Street drugs can cause severe damage to the skin. Inhaling solvents such as glue can permanently injure the delicate lining of the nasal cavity and cause sores to form around the nose and mouth. These sores may be the first clue that someone is trying these substances.

Injecting drugs with nonsterile needles can give rise to bacterial skin infections, abscesses, and cellulitis.

Jogger's nipple

Petroleum jelly applied to the nipples before jogging may prevent jogger's nipple, an eczema-like condition caused by friction from clothing combined with increased sweat levels. For women, a correctly fitting sports bra may help.

EXERCISE AND HOBBIES

Although exercise is obviously good for general health, it can generate a few problems as far as the skin and nails are concerned. Awareness of potential problems is the first step to avoiding them. In almost all cases, a few simple precautions are all you need to make sure that your exercise or hobby is not causing problems for your skin and nails.

Calluses and corns

For any sport, including walking, get good advice from an experienced person on the correct footwear, and be sure that shoes fit well. Badly fitting sport shoes can cause the formation of hard pads of skin that need careful treatment by a podiatrist.

Musician's neck

Fiddler's neck is a well-recognized skin problem found in professional violin and viola players. Friction from the chin rest can lead to a form of eczema and an acne-like cyst. In some cases, acne medication can be used to treat the condition; the cyst can be surgically removed.

Toenail dystrophy

It is important to be aware that when we run, walk fast, or dance, our feet go forward into the front of our shoes. This can lead to recurrent impact of the toe into the shoe, causing damage to the nail bed, where the nail is formed. The toenail can be severely thickened and misshapen. Prevention is better than cure, so ensuring that shoes fit well is a good first step. Anyone who is doing heavy manual work should wear shoes with steel toes.

Athlete's foot

Exercise causes increased perspiration, and this encourages the growth of fungus between the toes, in turn causing the condition known as athlete's foot. This can be prevented by wearing cotton socks and scrupulously drying your feet after exercise. OTC powders help ensure that feet are completely dry, and creams eradicate the fungus.

Medication and the skin

Almost any drug can cause a skin reaction, and many inflammatory skin diseases can be caused or made worse by drugs. Knowing about possible reactions can help you and your doctor pinpoint the likely culprit.

Some, but not all, drug reactions result from an allergy. Others are caused by overdose or the accumulation of a drug in the skin. Some are unwanted side effects of an otherwise useful drug. Some drugs are much more likely to cause skin reactions than others. Ask your doctor or pharmacist about possible side effects for your skin before taking any new drug. If you suddenly develop a skin problem soon after starting a new drug, ask your pharmacist whether it could be to blame and seek your doctor's advice on whether to continue taking it.

There are a number of well-defined skin reaction patterns associated with specific drugs.

RED ITCHY RASHES

The most common skin reactions to drugs are itchy, widespread, red bumpy rashes. In most cases, the rash erupts after a few days on the drug, but sometimes there is a delay of a few weeks. Stopping the drug usually makes the rash subside within a week. Drugs that commonly cause this rash include the antibiotic amoxicillin and NSAIDs.

URTICARIA AND ANAPHYLAXIS

Drugs may occasionally produce a severe allergic reaction within minutes of taking them, and this can be very serious. If you have had such a reaction in the past, you must carry an epinephrine injection for self-administration (commercially called an EpiPen, available with a prescription) and an alert bracelet or other notification. Drugs that may cause this reaction include aspirin, penicillin, morphine, and codeine.

ECZEMA

Contact dermatitis can be caused by the ingredients of topical creams and ointments. Lanolin, preservatives such as parabens, topical anesthetics, antihistamines, and antibiotics can all cause this reaction.

PHOTOTOXICITY

Some drugs increase the skin's sensitivity to the sun, so it can burn even on an overcast day. Examples of this are tetracycline antibiotics, oral contraceptives, and the thiazide drugs used for high blood pressure.

Drugs, topical or taken internally, and chemicals on the skin can interact with UV rays and cause immunological reactions—usually contact eczema. The eruption will only occur on areas of the body exposed to light such as the backs of the hands, the neck, nose, chin, and the forehead. This usually occurs after the second or third exposure to UV rays, and is often delayed by 2–3 weeks, so it can be difficult to work out the cause of these sorts of rashes.

HAIR LOSS

This commonly happens when people are given cytotoxic drugs to treat cancer. Hair nearly always regrows after treatment is over. Some drugs such as warfarin, antithyroid drugs, and the contraceptive pill can cause hair thinning.

SKIN PIGMENTATION CHANGES

Increased skin pigmentation may happen with photosensitivity, but some commonly used drugs can cause other types of pigment to be deposited in the skin. Minocycline, used to treat acne, may leave reversible blue deposits on scarred areas such as the face or shins.

SAFETY WITH HERBAL MEDICATIONS

Chinese herbs have proven successful in treating eczema and psoriasis in children. If you are going to try this treatment, doctors recommend buying the herbs from a reputable practitoner who uses only "standardized ingredients." If the ingredients are not standardized, you have no way of gauging how your body will react to them. Once a course of treatment is started, doctors recommend regular blood tests to monitor liver function.

Skin and hair care basics

Eating a balanced diet, drinking plenty of water, avoiding smoking and excess alcohol, exercising regularly, and getting enough sleep all contribute to healthy skin, especially when backed up by an effective skin-care routine.

Effective skin care should cleanse the skin regularly and replenish the moisture in its uppermost layers.

There are many skin care products on the market, and choosing what suits you can be a daunting prospect. You need to have a good idea what you are looking for before you start.

Skin care should also include protecting your skin against the harmful effects of ultraviolet (UV) rays by applying products that offer UV protection (see page 76).

Facial skin care for men
In the not too distant past, the concept of skin products especially for men seemed unthinkable. Today, ranges for men include cleansers, moisturizers, and astringents. The male skin needs at least as much care as female skin, perhaps more. Male skin is more prone to excessive oil production, so the regular use of deep-pore cleansers can help to keep the skin in optimum condition.

SKIN TYPES
Sebaceous skin glands—especially those on the forehead, and around the eyes, nose, and chin—produce sebum, a natural oil; the amount that is produced determines your skin type. If sebum fills the gaps between the dead surface cells, this results in a normal texture skin. If less oil is produced, the skin feels rougher; this is dry skin. If the glands are very active, the skin is oily; if this oil is only on the forehead, nose, and chin, this is called combination skin. Different skin types need different skin care routines (see panel below).

SOAPS AND FACE WASHES
Normal soaps contain detergents that are harsh on the skin and that reduce the amount of water and natural oils in its uppermost layers. This means that using soap and water on the face may leave the skin feeling tight and dry, particularly if you tend to have dry skin anyway. Alternative soaps and face washes that cleanse the skin without the use of detergents and contain moisturizers are available. For oily and spotty skin, medicated soaps and washes containing specially formulated gentle detergents can be beneficial.

DAILY CARE FOR THE FACE

Although skin-care regimens differ according to skin type, there are two basic steps that should be carried out by everyone: first, cleansing the skin of makeup, and second, moisturizing to help keep the skin supple and prevent moisture loss. Toning is not an essential part of skin care, but many people choose to use a toner to clear any residual makeup and freshen the skin before moisturizer is applied. In addition, exfoliation is considered a valuable measure for achieving healthy, glowing skin. Skin type can change through life, and a skin-care routine may need to be modified accordingly. For example, oily skin may develop at certain times in life, particularly during the teenage years, but may not be permanent— and skin generally becomes drier with age.

Normal skin
If you are one of those fortunate people who have normal skin, you still need to follow a daily skin-care regimen to ensure that it stays that way. Your skin should be thoroughly cleansed twice a day. Cleansers that are washed away with water are suitable and leave the skin feeling refreshed. Toners with alcohol should be avoided for normal skin; alcohol can dry the skin and leave it feeling tight and uncomfortable. Water-based moisturizing creams or lotions are perfect for normal skin, and are light and easily applied. The face can be exfoliated once a week to clear some of the dead cells on the surface. A mask can also be applied once a week. Various types of skin masks are available for normal skin and can be used in turn for a hydrating boost (a moisturizing mask) or for deeper cleansing (a clay mask).

SKIN CLEANSERS

Skin cleansers gently remove makeup and daily grime from the face without the use of harsh soaps. They can be used in place of soaps and are available in a number of forms, including creams and lotions that are applied to the skin and wiped off with a cottonball. Foaming washes are washed away with water, leaving the skin feeling refreshed. However, some people with dry skin find that even water can leave their face feeling tight and uncomfortable. If you are one of those people, you may find cleansing creams and lotions preferable.

TONER

A toner removes any remaining cleansing residue, closes pores, and returns the skin to its proper pH balance. The skin is then smooth and ready to absorb a moisturizer.

FACIAL SCRUBS

The small, smooth granules in facial scrubs remove dead cells from the skin surface (exfoliation), helping moisture enter and giving the skin a healthy glow. The scrub is rubbed over the face with gentle circular movements, avoiding the skin in the delicate eye area. This should be done no more than once a week.

The whole body can benefit from exfoliation. Body scrubs usually contain larger, slightly rougher granules than those found in facial scrubs. The body can be exfoliated two to three times a week.

FACE MASKS

These provide an intensive treatment, whether your skin needs a moisture boost, a deep cleansing, or a combination of the two. Masks are available in various forms, including thick creams and formulations designed to harden and then peel off. Leaving the mask on for a period of time means that the skin derives maximum benefit from the ingredients. Special eye masks are available to treat the delicate skin around the eyes. A weekly face mask treatment can benefit most skin types.

MOISTURIZERS

Applying moisturizer regularly is a vital part of skin care. These products are available in many different forms, and some are more effective than others.

What does a moisturizer do?

Moisturizers replenish the moisture and oils in the upper layers of the skin and provide a protective layer on the skin's surface to prevent moisture loss. Some moisturizers give protection against ultraviolet rays, reducing their damaging and aging

Oily skin

The skin should be cleansed twice a day with a face wash containing gentle detergents. If a toner is used, it should be formulated for oily skin; this can slightly reduce the natural oils (sebum), which are present in excess in oily skin. Even oily skin needs to be moisturized regularly. Water-soluble moisturizers that are light and easy to apply are usually preferable. The skin can be exfoliated and a deep cleansing clay mask applied once a week.

Dry skin

Dry skin products should contain ingredients that add and retain water in the skin's upper layers. Use a mild cleanser that contains no detergents, and if you use a toner, it should not contain alcohol. If you wash your face, the water should be warm, never hot. Moisturize twice daily with an intensive moisturizer.

Combination skin

Cleansers are available that are suited to combination skin. Cleansing can be followed by a mild toner applied to the oily areas. The whole face, including the oily parts, then needs to be moisturized. A water-based moisturizer will hydrate the dry cheeks adequately without making the oily central panel of the face more greasy. Extra moisture may sometimes be needed for the dry areas of the face. This can be achieved by applying a more intensive moisturizer rich in humectants. The face can be exfoliated gently once a week. Masks are available that are specially formulated to suit both dry and greasy skin. Alternatively, two masks may be used: clay for the oily areas and a moisturizing mask for dry patches.

Aloe vera gel is 90 percent water, so it is excellent for soothing and rehydrating the skin. Other ingredients include minerals, vitamins, enzymes, and amino acids.

effect on the skin. Everyone—but particularly people over age 30 and those with dry skin—should use a moisturizer with SPF 15 or higher every day.

A good moisturizer will make the skin feel softer and should relieve dryness without making the skin feel greasy. If you tend to have dry skin, the "tight" feeling should be relieved.

The skin of the face should be moisturized twice a day: in the morning to replenish moisture after washing or cleansing and especially at the end of the day when the face should be fully cleansed and a moisturizer applied.

Ideally, the body should be moisturized daily after a shower or bath, when the skin is still damp. Moisturizing the body twice a day is beneficial, particularly for those who have dry skin.

Which type should I use?

There are so many moisturizers available that it can be difficult to know which to choose, but you need to bear two things in mind: first, your skin type, and second, how much time you have available to care for it.

Creams tend to be the more intensive form of treatment. They are usually thick and for this reason may take a little longer to apply than more liquid products. Creams are often oil-based and are particularly suitable for skin that tends to be dry.

For normal and combination skin, lotions should provide adequate moisture. Lotions are light, easy to apply, and quick to dry. Some people with combination skin like to apply more intensive cream to the drier areas of their face, such as the cheeks, although combination skin products are made to suit all areas.

Gels are usually water-based and are particularly helpful for greasy or sensitive skin. They are light and easy to use and do not add extra oil that could overload the skin.

In addition, some moisturizers are available in two forms: day and night creams. For young people, it may be enough to use the same cream or lotion morning and night. Those over age 30 and people with dry skin may find it beneficial to use a thicker, more intensive treatment before bed.

HYPOALLERGENIC PRODUCTS

If you have sensitive skin, it is worth buying hypoallergenic products. These are made from highly purified ingredients and do not contain well-known allergens—ingredients that are known to be capable of causing

allergic reactions. However, "hypo" means "less," not "none:" Hypoallergenic products contain fewer potential irritants or allergens, not none at all. Some people find that plant-based hypoallergenic products cause fewer reactions on sensitive skin.

ANTIWRINKLE CREAMS

Many cosmetics companies claim that their moisturizers can halt the effects of time and actually reduce the appearance of fine lines and wrinkles. However, many of these products do little more than act as a kind of skin caulk, smoothing out the wrinkles by filling in the cracks between them. Other products contain AHAs (alphahydroxy acids), plant-derived ingredients that help to remove dead skin cells from the skin surface. As far as skin health is concerned, the important factor is not the appearance of lines but maintaining a sufficient moisture level in the skin.

BEFORE YOU BUY

When choosing a skin care product, it is worth reading the information on the label. Not only will this tell you whether the product is suitable for your skin type, it may also give valuable additional information, such as whether it gives UV protection.

If you are buying something for the first time, try the tester if one is available and then buy the smallest size possible. If you like the product, you can then invest in a larger economy size, and if you don't, you haven't wasted too much money.

BODY BRUSHING

Body brushing stimulates the blood circulation to the skin and improves skin tone. It is only suitable for the body because the skin of the face is too delicate. Body brushing treatment should be done in a warm room with the skin completely dry. A soft brush is swept firmly over the body, starting from the feet and working up. The brushing should be followed by moisturizing.

CARING FOR THE HANDS

The skin on the hands tends to age rapidly because it is frequently washed, comes into contact with all sort of substances, and is the skin most often exposed to damaging ultraviolet rays. In addition, the layer of natural oils protecting the back of the hand is thin, so moisture is easily lost. This makes moisturizing the hands an important part of skin care that may need to be done several times a day.

Moisturizers containing humectants such as glycerin replenish the moisture within the skin; petroleum jelly and other so-called occlusives reduce moisture loss. AHAs help remove the outer layer of dead cells and encourage the production of new skin cells.

In addition, massaging the hands when applying moisturizer increases the blood supply to the skin and so improves its condition. The nails also need attention and regular maintenance (see pages 63–64).

FEET AND FOOT CARE

Because our feet are hidden from view for most of the day, we tend to forget about them, but skin on the feet and particularly the heels is vulnerable to dryness and cracking. This tends to worsen as we get older.

Our feet are also prone to develop patches of hard skin. This can be reduced by wearing comfortable shoes that don't squash or pinch but support the foot.

Feet benefit from being washed and moisturized with foot lotion every day. Care should be taken when drying the feet—the skin between the toes needs to be dried thoroughly. Gently rubbing the skin with a foot file or pumice stone twice a week will reduce hard skin. Foot spas can relax tired feet and improve the condition of the skin—the warm water and the massaging effect increases the flow of blood to the skin. Soaking in a bowl of warm water can also relieve tired feet.

PROBLEM AREAS

The heels, elbows, and knees tend to get particularly dry and need special attention to prevent painful cracking. Gentle exfoliation with a body scrub every few days and massaging every day with a moisturizing cream that is rich in humectants will help keep the skin soft and supple. Fresh lemon juice applied with a cotton pad can also help soften the skin—these areas should then be washed and dried carefully.

CHOOSING DEODORANTS AND ANTIPERSPIRANTS

It is personal preference whether you choose a spray or a roll-on product. If you are prone to dryness and skin irritation, an unperfumed, hypoallergenic product is best. Many products also have hydrating properties to relieve dry skin. If you have very sensitive skin, it may take you a while to find a product that leaves your skin feeling comfortable and soft.

SKIN CARE FOR MEN

Skin products specially formulated to suit men's skin are available, and many men are now aware of the benefits of regular skin care.

Moisturizer can help keep the skin well-hydrated and supple. Men should consider using a moisturizer that offers UV protection, particularly when spending time outdoors.

Men tend to have larger skin pores, and when these become blocked with debris, blemishes can form. Pore cleansing strips gently peel away and remove blackheads without damaging the skin.

Aftershave acts as an astringent and toner for the skin. It helps return the skin to a slightly acidic state after the use of alkaline shaving creams. It also softens and smooths the skin by closing the pores.

SHAMPOOING YOUR HAIR

Hair can be washed daily without any problems as long as a few simple care rules are followed. Do not use very hot water, and when drying do not rub vigorously or use excessive heat. Poor-quality hair products are not good for hair and are a false economy.

It is best to let your hair dry naturally, but if you prefer to use a dryer, use a low setting only. Keep the dryer moving to prevent any damage to the hair shaft.

Let your hair hang naturally while you wash it. Stand in the shower or lean your head over the bath. Do not pile your hair onto the top of your head. This causes tangling and breakage.

Using warm water, rinse your hair thoroughly to prepare for shampooing.

tips for shampooing

While your hair is damp, loosen tangles with a wide-toothed comb. Taking a section of hair at a time, use gentle downward strokes. Start near the ends and work toward the roots, holding the hair just above the section you are combing to prevent dragging.

tips for drying

Do not apply shampoo directly to your hair from the bottle. Pour some into the palm of your hand.

Wrap a clean towel around your hair and pat dry using a blotting action. Do not rub vigorously—this will cause tangling and breakage.

Gently rub the shampoo between your palms. Starting at the scalp, work the shampoo into your hair gently with your fingers in a clawlike shape.

Leave the conditioner on for two minutes, and then rinse well.

tips for conditioning

Rinse your hair well to remove all traces of shampoo, allowing the water to cascade through the hair. Do not rub your wet hair.

Pour some conditioner into the palm of your hand, spread it between the palms, and then work it into your hair gently, evenly, and thoroughly.

HAIR CARE

Not only is there is a right way to shampoo and condition hair to keep it healthy, but different hair types respond to different treatments.

DRY, GREASY, OR NORMAL?

In addition to basic type—straight, wavy, or tightly curled (see page 44)—hair can be normal, dry or greasy. The quality and feel of hair change with age, stress, and trauma and also depend on how you treat the hair.

Dry hair

Dry hair does not shine and feels rough to the touch. It tangles easily, is prone to split ends and is difficult to style. This is because it does not contain enough moisture—the outer layer of the hair (the cuticle layer) has become porous so the inside of the hair (the cortex) cannot retain water. The condition is more common in longer hair than short, because the hair has been growing for longer and has been subjected to greater cosmetic and environmental trauma. In addition, chemical treatments such as perming, dyeing, and bleaching cause dryness. Dry hair should be treated with mild shampoos and conditioners. It also responds to intensive restructuring conditioners. These usually contain panthenol, which has a cumulative effect on the hair shaft, helping it to retain moisture and proteins, which help smooth the cuticle layer.

Greasy hair

The feel of the hair depends on the amount of grease present. Greasy hair tends to be limp, look flat, and have little volume. It soon gets greasy again after shampooing, because of a buildup of sebum

produced by the sebaceous glands in the scalp. Sebum is a natural oil that passes into the hair follicle and over the hair shaft. It does not penetrate the hair shaft but lies on its surface.

The amount of sebum produced by the body fluctuates: It is more abundant during puberty, for example, when there tends to be a higher level of male hormones present. It has been suggested that stress may increase the amount of sebum produced, as can poor-quality shampoos. It is not possible to keep the glands from producing sebum, nor does diet affect its production. The best course is to use a shampoo designed for greasy hair and wash hair daily, before too much grease has a chance to build up.

Normal hair

Normal hair is usually defined as hair that has not had any chemical applications and is neither greasy nor dry. The hair shines and is manageable; it looks good and healthy. To care for normal hair, use a mild shampoo and, if the hair is longer than 6 inches, perhaps a little conditioner from the middle to the ends, which will help soften environmental weathering.

SHAMPOOS AND CONDITIONERS

Shampoo produces lather, which aids the removal of dirt from the hair by trapping dirt particles and keeping them from being redeposited on the hair. For a shampoo to be effective, it must be able to remove grease and dirt from the hair without removing natural oils from the scalp. It must also be mild to avoid damaging the scalp, hair, or eyes.

Shampoos

The various components of shampoo each have a specific job.
- **Cleansing agents** remove grease and dirt from the hair. Two of the milder cleansing agents used are ammonium lauryl sulfate and ammonium laureth sulfate.
- **Hair-care additives** might include antidandruff agents, moisturizers, herbal extracts, and fruit extracts.
- **Functional additives** include preservatives, perfumes, colors, and pH controllers.

Conditioners

Most shampoos contain some conditioning agent, and this is usually sufficient for people with shorter, normal hair. For longer hair, hair that has been affected by environmental trauma, or hair that has been subjected to chemical applications or over-drying, more conditioning may be necessary to improve feel and manageability.

IT'S NOT TRUE!

"The more I wash my hair, the more greasy it becomes"

Washing hair frequently does not cause more oil to be produced. Irregular shampooing, however, will result in a buildup of grease as environmental dirt sticks to the oily surface of the hair, so it is best to wash greasy hair daily using a shampoo designed for greasy hair. Such shampoos are formulated to remove natural grease without damaging the hair shaft.

Conditioners help smooth the outside layer (the cuticle) of the hair and reduce static electricity, which causes "fly-away" hair. They may also contain panthenol and silicones, which increase the moisture-holding properties of the hair and smooth the hair shaft. This reduces tangling and makes the hair softer. Conditioner leaves hair easier to comb when wet or dry, which is immensely important for dry, permed, bleached, or dyed hair.

Home treatment can also be applied using vegetable oil. Almond, corn, and sunflower are all light oils that are easy to remove from the hair by shampooing. Pour 3 ounces of oil into a suitable container and warm gently until lukewarm. Apply to the hair, massage, and leave for 30 minutes. Remove the oil using a mild shampoo in the normal way. This can be done two to three times weekly.

Product buildup

Some hair products cause a gradual buildup of residue on the hair, making it look dull and limp. This can be avoided by regularly changing your hair products or by using an antiresidue shampoo once a week.

COMMON PROBLEMS

The two most common problems affecting hair are dandruff and head lice. Dandruff affects people of any hair type at any time. Head lice can affect anyone but are more common among school children.

Dandruff

This is a problem caused by flaking of the top layer of skin on the scalp. This flaking occurs all over the body, all of the time: Millions of tiny flakes are lost every day. The purpose of this is to remove skin bacteria, keeping the number on the skin to a minimum. On the scalp, the hair can trap these flakes, and they build up or accumulate into larger flakes. The damp warm conditions that result are favorable to the multiplication of bacteria and yeasts and can exacerbate the problem.

The best way to control dandruff is by using a shampoo containing zinc pyrithione. Use daily and leave on the scalp for 2 to 3 minutes before rinsing. If the treatment is ineffective after two weeks, it is best to visit your doctor.

HEAD LICE

There are more between 6 and 12 million cases of head lice in the United States every year. Head lice are highly contagious and if one person in a family becomes infected, everyone in the household must be treated.

There are five things you should know about lice and nits:
- Lice are the insects, and nits are the eggs.
- It is impossible to drown lice.
- Nits are harder to eliminate than lice. This is why treatment should not be interrupted.
- Nits should not be confused with dandruff. Nits are stuck to the hair, and dandruff flakes off.
- Empty eggs are white. Live eggs are the same colour as the hair and so are harder to see.

Nearly all lice treatments are available over the counter. A single application will usually kill all head lice, taking about 12 hours to clear the problem. A second application is necessary 10 days later to kill any newly hatched nits.

Alcohol-based pesticide solutions are the most effective, but water-based alternatives are available for small children and eczema or asthma sufferers. Problems arising from overuse are only likely if manufacturer's instructions are not followed correctly.

Alternative lice treatments

For those with concerns about using pesticides on children's heads, there are alternative methods for getting rid of lice (some are shown at right). They are as effective as chemical methods, but tend to be more time-consuming.

Do combined shampoos and conditioners work?

Combined shampoos and conditioners are extremely convenient: They save on storage space and time and are useful products to take traveling. They are not particularly effective for cleaning the hair, however.

When a normal shampoo is lathered on wet hair, it lifts the dirt and grime from the follicles. When the lather is rinsed, the dirt is rinsed away. It is only after the hair has been cleaned properly that it is ready to be conditioned.

Combined shampoos and conditioners might make your hair feel conditioned, but that is deceptive. The chemical producing the effect is building a waxy coating over the follicles that will eventually make them look dull. It is best not to use these products on a regular basis.

ASK THE EXPERT?

Aromatherapy oils

Many oils, including eucalyptus, geranium, parsley, Scotch pine, rosemary, lavender, thyme, and tea tree, will kill lice. The safest to use on children are tea tree and lavender.

In a small bottle mix 1 tsp pure tea tree or lavender essential oil, with 5 tbsp warm water, 2 tbsp pure alcohol or vodka and 1 tsp castor oil. Shake the bottle well, then make a series of ½ in. partings in the hair. Apply the lotion over the scalp covering approximately 2 in. up the hair shaft from the roots and leave for 12 hours or overnight. Shampoo using warm water, massaging well into the scalp. Rinse and repeat. Comb through the hair with a nit comb to remove dead lice and egg cases. If possible, leave hair to dry naturally—heat will evaporate the active ingredients. Repeat every three days for two weeks and check regularly for any reinfestation. Swimming pool chlorine, perms, and hair dyeing can reduce the effectiveness of the treatment.

Bug Buster kit

Available in the U.K. from all good pharmacies, this is a special comb that is used on wet hair that has been coated with conditioner. The slippery surface makes the lice slower moving and unable to grip the scalp, so the comb can hook them out. Six bug-busting sessions over a two-week period should clear the problem. Unlike with chemical treatments, lice cannot become resistant to bug busting.

Electronic comb

This battery-powered comb has a tiny sensor on the tip of each tooth. It can hardly be felt by humans but as soon as the sensor touches a head louse, an electric current is released that kills it. The dead lice are caught in the teeth of the comb and are easily removed. Because the comb does not kill the eggs, it is necessary to repeat the treatment every two days for two weeks. Electronic combs are difficult to use—and therefore less successful—on long hair.

CUTTING HAIR

Human hair does not grow at the same rate throughout the scalp. Some hairs will be in the middle of a growing phase, whereas others are coming to the end of their phase, when growth is slower. This means that hair will start to look a little untidy again about 6 to 8 weeks after a haircut, and it's time to revisit your hair stylist.

If you are in the process of growing your hair long, it will still need a trim every two months to clean up the ends. In two months your hair grows an average of 1 inch. If you do not want to lose all the growth you have gained between cuts, your hairdresser should remove no more than ½ inch.

When to cut a baby's hair

Baby hair is very fine and soon starts to look a little "ragged." If the ends are trimmed every 6 to 8 weeks it will keep the hair looking neat. There's no right or wrong time for a baby to have a first hair cut, but hair should be trimmed before it gets near the baby's eyes.

CHOOSING A HAIRBRUSH

A well-made brush should last for many years. All brushes should have even tufts or rows of bristles to allow loose, shed hairs to collect in the grooves without interfering with the action of the brush.

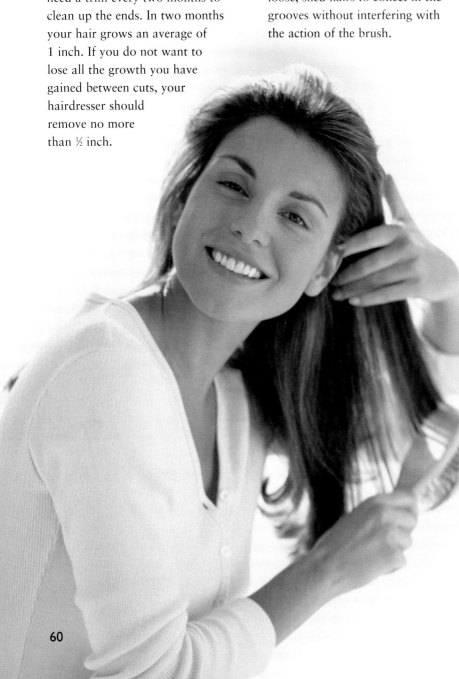

There are many types of hairbrushes available, and they fall into two main categories—those for everyday brushing and those for styling.

A natural bristle is recommended for general use because it has a gentler action and redistributes the natural hair oils evenly.

For styling—usually done using a hair dryer—brushes tend to be made of nylon. It is best to choose a brush with rounded nylon ball tips that are molded as part of the bristle and not just attached to the top, because they easily break off. Using a brush that is missing the nylon ball tips can scratch the scalp or damage the hair.

Thick coarse hair can benefit from using a paddle brush, which can create a smooth look and style. If you have wavy hair, look for a round vented brush. To avoid frizziness, curly hair should be "brushed" with a wide-tooth comb, and a vented brush with natural bristles is ideal for thin, fine hair. Long hair should be untangled with a wide-tooth comb, before being styled.

To clean your brush, use a comb to remove built up hair. Soak the brush in hot water and a few drops of shampoo. Rinse and dry thoroughly.

Brushing your hair

Always start brushing in sections from the ends of the hair working up to the roots. Hold the mesh of hair just above the section being brushed. This reduces tension on the hair strands and will prevent breakage.

100 strokes a night?

Women used to brush their hair 100 times every night to remove dirt and disperse natural oils. This is no longer necessary, but it can still be beneficial: Use a natural bristle brush and brush deeply from the scalp.

Body hair

As mammals, all human beings have body hair. The amount varies with genetic background and age—whether it is too much or too little is a matter of personal perception and social norms.

The amount of body hair in some areas is a major source of concern for many people, who can spend significant amounts of time and money trying to remove it.

REMOVING UNWANTED HAIR

The most common methods of hair removal fall into two categories:

- **Epilation** This means that the hair is removed below the surface of the skin and refers to the complete removal of the hair from the follicle. This can be done by plucking and waxing.
- **Depilation** This is removal at skin level, either by chemically damaging the hairs so that they break off or by shaving.

Epilation

Waxing and plucking are painful but successful ways of removing hair. The effect is temporary (usually no more than 6 weeks, and often considerably less) because the follicle continues to produce new hair cells. Repeated removal of hairs can cause disruption of the anatomy of the hair-growing area and lead to the formation of ingrown hairs and inflammation of the follicles (folliculitis). These conditions are difficult to treat.

Plucking is viable for small areas, but it is too painful and time-consuming for larger areas. Plucking is ideal for any stray hairs, but avoid over-plucking eyebrows, because the hairs may not grow back.

Wax can be applied hot or cold and is a home or salon treatment. It involves the application of wax to areas of unwanted hair. After the wax hardens, it is pulled off the skin, along with the embedded hairs. Generally, waxing done by someone else is more successful than self-administered waxing—partly because of training, but also because many people find it hard to inflict discomfort on themselves.

Depilation

If epilation seems too uncomfortable, depilatory cream may be the answer. Again, this is a temporary solution, because the hair follicle is not being damaged and hair will regrow. Depilation creams are easy to apply and work by removing hair just below the surface of the skin. They contain sodium thioglycolate and calcium thioglycolate, which dissolve the keratin chemically. The mixture of chemicals produces an unpleasant odor, but this goes away after rinsing. The disadvantages are that the effect is shortlived, often less than a week, and the chemicals can irritate the skin. They should not be used on sensitive areas such as the face, and if a cream is being used for the first time, it should be patch tested first to avoid an adverse reaction.

Before applying the cream, wash the area with a warm washcloth to soften the hairs and open the follicles

LASER HAIR REMOVAL

Laser hair removal works by pulsing a laser for a millisecond, emitting a beam of light onto the skin. The light energy passes harmlessly through the skin but is absorbed by the pigment in the hair follicle and hair shaft. By absorbing this laser energy, the hair follicles are disabled, impairing their ability to grow.

Treatment is described as being a little uncomfortable—a tingling, stinging sensation. Because some areas of the body are more sensitive than others, topical anesthetic may be applied before treatment to lessen discomfort. The treatment time depends on the area: The upper lip takes only a few minutes but the back or legs can take up to an hour.

Laser hair removal works best on people with fair skin and dark hair: Blonde, gray and white hairs do not respond well, although a lot depends on the skill of the practitioner you choose. Treatments are scheduled to coincide with hair follicles being in an active growth phase—which is every 4 to 8 weeks. Laser hair removal is often called "permanent"; most people lose up to 70 percent of hair after three to five treatments.

so the cream will penetrate better. An effective chemical depilatory will damage the skin as well as the hair, but in normal healthy skin this does not usually cause a problem. Do not leave the cream on longer than recommended.

Shaving

Shaving is even faster than using a depilatory cream. Women have the same choices as men in terms of wet or dry shaving; both are equally fast and efficient.

- **Wet shaving** Although more time-consuming, this causes fewer problems with dry skin and chafing than dry shaving. Modern shaving creams contain moisturizers, and the action of rubbing in cream tones the skin. In ancient times, oil was used to soften the beard prior to shaving, and this method has been reintroduced recently. Wet shaving provides the closest shave.

- **Dry shaving** The obvious advantage of the dry shave is that it dispenses with the need for hot water and shaving cream, allowing shaving to be cleaner, safer, and more mobile. Electric shavers make it virtually impossible to cut yourself. Dry shaving typically does not produce as close a shave as wet shaving.

Different areas of the body should be shaved in different directions:

- The face should be shaved first in the direction of hair growth and then against.
- Legs should be shaved in an upward direction, against the direction of hair growth.
- Underarm hair grows in different directions, so this area should be shaved down, up, and then across for the closest shave.
- Bikini area skin is very delicate, so hair should be shaved in the same direction as hair growth to prevent irritation.

FEMALE FACIAL HAIR

For many women, excessive or over-dark facial hair is a particular cause of embarrassment and concern. A number of treatments, both temporary and permanent, are available.

Bleaching the hair with diluted hydrogen peroxide and ammonia solution is a safe and simple way of disguising hair growth. If using a product for the first time, always patch test your skin beforehand. Shaving should be avoided in this area because it can leave unsightly stubble. However, waxing is effective, leaving the skin clean and smooth. It is best to visit a professional for this.

In skilled hands, electrolysis and short-wave diathermy can successfully destroy individual hairs. Electrolysis is a long process and can cause local pain. Unwanted effects may be pitted scars and postinflammatory hyperpigmentation (PIHP). Regrowth occurs, but gradually the hairs become thinner and paler. It is vital to find a reputable practitioner: Poorly done electrolysis can cause scarring.

UNWANTED MALE NOSE AND EAR HAIR

It is thought that the male hormone reponsible for baldness may also be linked to nasal and ear hair growth—as men get older this hair becomes longer and coarser. Ear and nose hair can be easily trimmed, but it should never be plucked, because this can tear the delicate skin and cause an infection. The safest method is to use a specially designed electric trimmer.

Smooth operator
To avoid prolonging the localized pain of waxing, strips should be pulled upward quickly, in a single motion.

Healthy and good-looking nails

Many of us do not give our nails a lot of thought. However, because they protect our fingers and toes and enhance our touch and fine motor skills, their health is extremely important.

NORMAL NAIL GROWTH

Fingernails grow at a rate of about .004 inch per day and are replaced approximately every 4 to 6 months. Toenails grow more slowly and can take up to twice as long to replace themselves. How quickly and how well they grow depends on several factors: age, hormones, time of year (they grow faster in the summer), infections, nutrition, and trauma.

Each nail rises up from a nail root made up of the normal layers of cells in the skin. The outer layer forms the cuticle, and the nail itself rests on what is called the nail bed. The nail bed supports the nail as it grows outward from the nail matrix. It normally reaches the end of the nail bed and extends beyond it: When it does so, this section is termed the free edge.

WHY NAILS BREAK

Nails can break, tear, or split for many different reasons. The most common reason is having the nails submerged in water and detergents too much. It is important to protect the nails from excessive moisture—this can cause splitting and peeling. The easy answer to this is to wear household gloves while doing chores, especially cleaning and gardening. Try to avoid nail damage—don't use your nails as tools for prying things open, and watch out for closing doors. It pays to take care.

If you know that this is not a major factor in your case, then check out your diet and lifestyle (see page 72). You might be lacking in nutrients that will not only benefit your nails but will also do wonders for your skin and hair.

HOW TO CUT NAILS

The best time for cutting your nails is after a bath, when your nails are softer and thus easier to cut. This is particularly the case with toenails.

Helping hands
It is important to protect the skin on the hands because it has extensive contact with cleaning agents and environmental hazards.

A proper nail clipper will take most of the effort out of cutting and is more controllable than scissors.

Be careful not to cut your nails too short—this can expose extremely sensitive skin normally protected by the nail. After cutting, use a simple emery board to even them out, always filing in one direction for the smoothest effect.

Similarly, don't cut toenails too short. Cut them straight across to prevent ingrown toenails. Smooth them off so that they do not scratch your skin or get caught—or make holes—in your socks or stockings.

If you find bending over to be a problem, either from a sore hip or pregnancy, there are long-handled toenail clippers on the market that will make the job much easier.

Do nail strengtheners work?

Nail strengtheners do make nails harder, but there are a couple of things to bear in mind. They seem to work best when you use them for relatively short periods of time. Experts recommend you do not use them for any longer than 6 to 8 weeks at a time. Continuous use will over-harden your nails, making them brittle, so that you have turned one nail problem into another.

When choosing a nail strengthener, be sure to get a product that does not contain formaldehyde; this toxic substance was once widely used but has now been superseded by safer ingredients. Take extra care during pregnancy: If you have any doubts about a product's safety, don't use it.

ASK THE EXPERT

GIVE YOURSELF A MANICURE
You will need
- *a bowl of warm water*
- *nail clippers*
- *emery board*
- *cuticle pusher (wooden or plastic, or use a cotton swab)*
- *scrub cream*
- *hand cream*

Wash your hands and clean out any dirt under your fingernails. Then soak your nails in warm water for about 5 minutes; this will soften both the nails and cuticles.

Clip your nails to the desired length and shape, finishing by filing them to smooth the edge. Be sure to file in one direction only to "seal" the edge instead of roughening it.

Gently push back the cuticle. Do not damage the cuticles—they protect the nail bed from trauma and bacteria. Only cut a piece of cuticle away if it is in danger of tearing.

Take a generous amount of scrub cream (a facial one is fine) and massage this into your hands for a few minutes. This will remove any dead skin cells. Rinse well to leave rosy, smooth skin.

Thoroughly dry your hands and then apply hand cream, making sure you don't forget to massage it into the cuticles to keep them supple and to prevent them from cracking.

Cutting babies' nails

It can be daunting cutting an infant's nails. Because a baby's nails are so soft, however, you may find that they flake away all by themselves. A lot of parents nibble off tiny nails to prevent having to use clippers or scissors on them. Once this becomes too difficult, do what you would do yourself. Wait until after a bath and use small nail clippers to cut away any nails that are too long and may be causing self-inflicted scratches. Try to prevent cutting away too much, as this will only cause discomfort to the baby, especially if the nail becomes infected. Trimming little and often is the best option.

NAIL CONDITION

Nails in poor condition can be a result of dietary deficiencies (see page 72). A crash diet or a strict vegan lifestyle can also affect nail health. Contrary to popular belief, white spots on the nails have nothing to do with calcium deficiency; they are simply little air pockets under the surface, usually caused by minor traumas to the nail.

Vertical ridges on nails are a normal sign of aging that start to occur in middle age. They can't be prevented, but they can be smoothed out by buffing. Horizontal ridges, also known as "Beau's lines," are caused by an interruption in the growth of the nail because of recent illness, severe stress, or injury to the nail. These ridges grow out in time.

FOOD AND DRINK FOR SKIN, HAIR, AND NAILS

So much of our appearance is determined by our internal health. For glowing skin, shiny hair, and strong nails, your diet needs to contain a range of essential nutrients, particularly those that contribute to the structure of collagen in the skin and keratin in the nails and hair.

 66 *For overall nail, skin, and hair health, every meal should be nutritious and well-balanced. Here are some meal ideas to try.*

 68 *The skin directly reflects our health. These are the essential vitamins or minerals you need to keep dull and tired looking skin at bay.*

 71 *Shiny hair and strong nails depend on a good supply of iron, zinc, and calcium: The best sources of these nutrients are described here.*

Eating plan for healthy skin, hair, and nails

A diet consisting of fresh, unprocessed foods is vital for the health of your entire body, not just your skin. Try to include plenty of fresh fruit and vegetables and foods with high levels of essential fatty acids.

Breakfast
1 bowl of muesli with
   lowfat milk, topped with
   a tablespoon of flax seeds and
   a handful of raspberries
1 cup of herbal tea
   OR
half a grapefruit
1 container of lowfat yogurt topped
   with a tablespoon of flax seeds
1 slice of toast with 1 tsp lowfat
   spread and 1 tsp yeast extract
1 cup of herbal tea

Lunch
Grilled chicken breast served with
   young leaf spinach salad with tofu
   dressing, and focaccia bread
Sliced mango
Glass of water or calcium-fortified
   soy milk

   OR
1 serving of smoked salmon served
   with a potato salad made using
   lowfat yogurt and Dijon mustard,
   and a serving of cherry tomatoes
Orange and date salad
Glass of water or orange juice

Flax seeds are a rich source of essential fatty acids including omega-3, 6, and 9.

Dinner

Pan-seared salmon fillet served with baked sweet potatoes and stir-fried zucchini and mixed peppers.

Mixed fruit salad topped with yogurt

1 cup of green tea

OR

Grilled pork chop served with apple sauce, homemade gravy, blanched broccoli and carrots, and mashed potatoes

Baked apple with a handful of raisins, served with homemade custard made using skim milk

1 cup of herbal tea

Snacks

A handful of pumpkin seeds

Raw vegetables with lowfat hummus

Unlimited fruit

Rye bread topped with lowfat cream cheese and sliced pineapple

Remember to drink plenty of water throughout the day to prevent dehydration.

How foods affect the skin

Just as foods can affect energy levels, they can also affect appearance. A balanced intake of nutrients will contribute to your health on the inside and will be reflected on the outside in clear skin, healthy hair, and strong nails.

NUTRIENTS FOR HEALTHY SKIN

The most important vitamins and minerals for the health of your skin are vitamin A, the B vitamins, vitamin C, vitamin E, and zinc.

Vitamin A

Vitamin A helps maintain the structural integrity of skin cells. A deficiency disturbs the delicate balance of the skin and results in the loss of cells that produce lubricants to keep the skin soft and supple. This in turn leads to infection, irritation, and sloughing off of the surface of the skin.

Everyday foods contain two forms of vitamin A: retinol, which is derived from animal products, and carotenes (mostly beta-carotene), which can be found in fruit and vegetables. The best sources of retinol are liver, fish liver oils, kidneys, dairy foods, and eggs. Beta-carotene is found mainly in carrots and dark green, yellow, or orange vegetables. The darker the vegetable, the more beta-carotene it contains. The recommended daily intake (RDI) of vitamin A is 700 micrograms for a man and 600 micrograms for a woman. A glass of carrot juice or a 90-gram serving of spinach provides the daily amount; a serving of liver or liver pâté exceeds it at least fourfold.

B-group vitamins

Niacin is a B vitamin, and niacin deficiency has been linked to a disease called pellagra. Symptoms include dermatitis, in which the skin becomes dark and scaly—especially when exposed to light—as well as diarrhea and dementia. Although it is rare to develop a deficiency in the

Skin-smart diet
The first step toward a better complexion is to ensure that you are not missing vital nutrients in your diet. Fruit and vegetables are packed with skin-boosting vitamins and minerals.

VITAMIN A CONTENT OF SELECTED FOODS

	Portion size (g)	Vitamin A (µg)		Portion size (g)	Vitamin A (µg)
Liver, calf, fried	100	25200	Spinach, boiled	90	576
Liver, pig, stewed	100	22600	Kale	95	534
Liver, lamb, fried	100	19700	Mango	140	450
Liver, chicken, fried	100	10500	Carrots, young, boiled	60	443
Liver pâté	40	2960	Spring greens, boiled	95	359
Sweet potato, baked	130	1112	Butternut squash, baked	65	354
Carrots, old, boiled	60	756	Cantaloupe	100	322
Carrot juice	60	678	Papaya	140	189
Swiss chard, boiled	50	655	Savoy cabbage, boiled	95	100

U.S., it makes sense to ensure an adequate amount in the diet. The U.S. RDI for niacin is 13 to 18 milligrams for adults and 9 to 13 for children. Good sources include meat, potatoes, bread, and fortified breakfast cereals.

Deficiency of B-group vitamins riboflavin (vitamin B_2) and pyridoxine (vitamin B_6) cause skin lesions or sores, especially at the corners of the mouth, eyelids, and genital areas. Deficiency is rare unless the diet is short on milk, meat, fortified cereal products and eggs. The RDIs for riboflavin and pyridoxine are 1.7 milligrams and 2 milligrams, respectively, for all adults.

The B-group vitamin biotin is needed in small amounts by the body to break down fat. A rich source is egg yolk, and smaller amounts are found in milk and dairy products, cereals, fish, yeast, fruit, and vegetables. Biotin deficiency is rare. It can occur if excessive amounts of raw egg white are consumed. Raw egg white contains the compound avidin, which attaches or binds itself to biotin making it unavailable to the body for absorption. In such cases, deficiency leads to a dry scaly dermatitis.

Vitamin C

Vitamin C is an important antioxidant that helps maintain healthy tissues and fight wrinkles. It also plays an important role in the formation of collagen in the skin. A deficiency results in bleeding, especially from blood vessels underneath the surface of the skin and the gums. The best sources include citrus fruits, potatoes, peppers, cabbage, and eggplant. The RDI is 60 milligrams for all adults.

Vitamin E

Vitamin E is another important antioxidant for healthy skin. It helps maintain the structural integrity of cell membranes. This vitamin is found in many foods and, because it is fat soluble, can be stored in the body, so deficiency is rare. The richest sources are vegetable oils, nuts and seeds, some cereal products, and egg yolk. The RDI is 8 to 10 milligrams per adult—cooking with 1 tablespoon of sunflower oil and eating a handful of hazelnuts provides the daily requirement.

Zinc

Zinc works with vitamin C to make healthy collagen—an essential component of connective tissues. The total amount of zinc in the adult body has been estimated to be about 1.4 to 2.3 grams, of which 20 percent is in the skin. A deficiency can lead to weeping dermatitis around the body orifices and on the extremities such as hands and feet, eczema, poor wound healing, and reduced immune system function. Zinc deficiency has also been shown to worsen preexisting acne. Oysters, pumpkin seeds, pecan nuts, red meat, whole wheat, and rye flour are all good sources. The U.S. RDI is 15 milligram per day for adults.

Essential fatty acids (EFAs)

Some types of polyunsaturated fat are deemed essential because they must be derived from the diet—the body cannot make them from other polyunsaturated fats. These EFAs are called omega-3 and omega-6 fats, and they help hydrate the skin and increase its moisture content. A deficiency of EFAs can result in a scaly rash because water loss from the skin increases. Topical

Do EFAs offer relief from eczema and psoriasis?

The incidence of atopic eczema has been rising over the past decade. Many hypotheses have been suggested, including a decline in breastfeeding and a deficiency of essential fatty acids (EFAs). Studies have shown conflicting results; some have concluded that breastfeeding prevents atopic eczema, but others have found no evidence. Similarly with EFAs, trials using fish oil as a dietary supplement for atopic eczema have shown conflicting results, although the EFA linoleic acid (found in evening primrose oil and starfruit oil) has been shown to be beneficial for eczema. The effect of EFAs on psoriasis appears to be more positive. A number of trials using fish oil supplements to treat psoriasis showed positive results, but again these are inconclusive.

ASK THE EXPERT

applications on the skin have been shown to reverse these symptoms.

Good sources of EFAs include oily fish, vegetables, and red meat. There is not yet an RDI for EFAs, but many doctors recommend 0.65 gram of omega-3 (no less than 0.2 gram) and 4.4 grams of omega-6 per day. Flax seeds (and flax seed oil) are also good sources of EFAs. Flax seeds can be sprinkled on salads and cooked vegetables or combined with flour to make breads and pancakes. Flaxseed oil comes in an edible form and, like olive and rapeseed oils, is high in unsaturated fats, which is heart healthy. It also contains lignans, which have anticancer properties.

FOOD ALLERGIES

The immune system protects the body from harmful foreign proteins called antigens by generating a response to get rid of them. Antibodies are produced to specifically bind with the antigen to deactivate and eliminate it. In food allergies, an individual's immune system reacts in this way to a food that has no harmful effect in the majority of people.

Signs and symptoms of food allergies vary from person to person. There are different types of reactions. One of the most common involves the production of histamine, which can cause a number of symptoms including urticaria or skin rashes. In some individuals, such allergies have been linked to the consumption of

milk, eggs, fish, shellfish, nuts, and strawberries, and if any one of these is implicated, exclusion of that food is advised. This type of allergy arises in early childhood and appears to trigger abnormal inflammatory processes in the skin that are chronic and recurrent.

DIGESTION AND THE SKIN

An important aspect of skin health is a healthy colon and digestive process. If the colon is not moving food efficiently or if the liver or kidneys are struggling to process waste, toxins may build up in the bloodstream. This may have an impact on the appearance of the skin.

To aid the proper functioning of the digestive system, it is important to get plenty of fiber in your diet. You should also limit the amount of processed foods and sugars in your diet and limit alcohol intake. A well-balanced diet goes a long way in maintaining skin health. Many people find that drinking a cup of warm water with a squeeze of fresh lemon juice first thing in the morning helps flush out toxins, and herbalists recommend milk thistle supplements to help cleanse the liver and improve skin health.

Drink your way to skin health
Drinking more water could be the simple tonic your skin needs. Water acts as an internal moisturizer, promoting clearer skin and a glowing complexion.

WATER—VITAL FOR SKIN HEALTH

Water is essential for life; it makes up about two thirds of body weight and is vital for regulating body fluids. The average adult should consume 2.5 quarts of water a day. This will ensure that you avoid dehydration, which can lead to dull, lifeless, dry skin.

MALNUTRITION

Although rarely seen in Westernized countries, malnutrition can lead to a skin condition in which a sequence of changes similar to sunburn occur. The skin becomes darker, with the outer skin becoming dry and thin, and is easily split and ulcerated.

Foods for healthy hair and nails

Eat a well-balanced diet for the general good health of your hair and nails, with particular emphasis on maintaining iron, calcium, and zinc levels. Dietary deficiency is one among several different causes of hair loss and problem nails.

IRON

Better known for keeping blood in good health, iron also has an effect on the condition of your hair. General hair loss has been linked to low iron levels, which means that women who have heavy periods and those who eat little or no red meat have an increased risk of hair loss.

To maximize iron absorption, various dietary factors should be considered when preparing meals.

- Consuming vitamin C-rich foods such as fruits, vegetables, and juice with a meal will double or triple the amount of iron absorbed from nonmeat or fish sources.
- Protein-rich foods such as meat, fish, and seafood promote the absorption of iron.

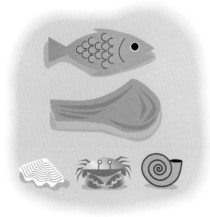

- Fermented products such as soy sauce enhance the absorption of iron from nonmeat or fish sources.
- Phytate and fiber-rich foods such as cereals, bran, seeds, and nuts inhibit the absorption of iron.
- Tea, coffee, cocoa, spinach, and spices contain compounds called phenols that inhibit iron absorption from legumes, cereals, and vegetables.
- Calcium-rich foods such as milk and cheese interfere with the absorption of iron in a meal.

To optimize iron levels or to replenish your body's stores, include iron-rich foods in your diet. The best sources are red meat—especially liver—egg yolks, dried fruit, fortified breakfast cereals, and green leafy vegetables. Then, to maximize iron absorption, eat these foods together with those that are high in vitamins. For example, have a glass of orange juice with your meal. Try not to drink tea or coffee for at least half an hour after a meal to minimize the adverse effects of tea, coffee, and milk on iron absorption.

Our requirements for iron vary throughout our lives: The RDI for infants up to 6 months old is 6 milligrams; for those up to 1 year old and adult men, it is 10 milligrams. Women and adolescent girls need 15 milligrams per day, 30 during pregnancy.

THE NEED FOR ZINC

Zinc is an essential component of hair—scalp hair in children has been estimated to contain 125 to 225 micrograms zinc per gram of hair. In some studies, zinc deficiency has been shown to lead to hair loss, excessive fragility of hair, sparse scalp hair, and absent pubic hair. Zinc deficiency has been shown to be the cause of hair loss in the disease acrodermatitis enteropathica, which is characterized by alopecia as well as diarrhea and dermatitis. Hair is lost diffusely and extensively and existing hair lacks pigment, making it fragile and prone to excessive breakage.

Although zinc can be found in a wide variety of foods, its absorption by the body depends on the composition of the diet. The risk of zinc deficiency is highest when the diet contains large quantities of unrefined cereals and little animal protein.

- **Phytates** in whole-grain cereals, legumes, and other vegetables bind to zinc, making it unavailable for absorption by the body.
- **Animal protein** improves the absorption of zinc from foods.
- **Essential fatty acid (EFA)** deficiency has been shown to cause hair loss. EFAs form two groups—omega-3 and omega-6 fats—and can be found in oily fish, as well as in vegetables and red meat.

MALNUTRITION

Malnutrition can have a very serious effect on hair, weakening its attachment to the skin so that it falls out easily and painlessly. Remaining hair becomes thin and straight and may turn gray. Patients can go completely bald, although this is usually reversible.

FOODS FOR HEALTHY NAILS

Nails are a type of skin made up mainly of the protein keratin. They grow at the rate of about .002 to .05 inch per week. Our nails reveal a great deal about the state of our health. There are numerous vitamins and minerals that are specifically needed by the body to make healthy and strong nails, so deficiencies over a period of time will have a detrimental effect.

Iron is essential for the maintenance of healthy cells, and a long-term deficiency can cause nails to become spoon-shaped, brittle, and thin. Two sources of iron—hem and nonhem—can be found in our foods, and there are various ways of making sure iron is absorbed when we eat (see page 71).

Very small amounts of the B-group vitamin biotin are needed for the formation of strong nails. This can be produced by the bacteria that live in our large intestine. Rich sources include egg yolk, milk, and dairy products, liver and other organ meats, soy products, and yeast.

Calcium is the most abundant mineral in the body, with about 99 percent of it in the bones, teeth, and nails. When bound together with phosphorous, calcium strengthens the skeleton. Few foods besides milk, yogurt, cheese, most breads, calcium-fortified soy milk, tofu, green leafy vegetables, and hard water contain significant amounts of calcium.

The RDI for calcium for an adult is 1100 milligrams a day, which is achieved, for example, by eating a container of yogurt, a small chunk of cheese, and a serving of young leaf spinach. Breastfeeding mothers require an additional 500 milligrams a day. To meet this, add a serving of tofu and a slice of white bread, for example, or a serving of canned sardines with bones and a handful of raisins.

CALCIUM CONTENT OF SELECTED FOODS

	Portion	Calcium (mg)
Sardines with bones, canned in salt water	140 g	540
Whole-milk yogurt	150 g	300
Cheddar cheese	40 g	288
Lowfat yogurt	150 g	285
Cheddar cheese, vegetarian	40 g	276
Lowfat or skim milk	150 ml	175
Whole milk	150 ml	168
Brie cheese	50 g	92
Ice cream, dairy	125 g	90
Baked beans, canned in tomato sauce	135 g	65
White bread	36 g	40
Watercress	20 g	34
White rice, boiled	180 g	32
Boiled egg	50 g	29
Cabbage, white, boiled	95 g	25
Peanuts, dry roasted	40 g	21
Zucchini, boiled	100 g	19
Whole-grain bread	36 g	19
Raisins	18 g	12
Braising steak, stewed	140 g	11
Potatoes, boiled	175 g	9
Apples	100 g	4
Cod, baked	120 g	3

THE WEATHER AND YOUR SKIN

Most people are now aware that despite the good things the sun can do for skin and general health, it can also cause damage if we do not take precautions. Other weather factors such as wind, rain, and snow may also have an impact on our skin, hair, and nails.

Safety in the sun is of paramount importance for everyone, especially children, to keep skin young-looking and free from disease.

In some circumstances, winter can pose as many risks to skin health as summer does. Find out how to minimize the impact of each.

How the sun affects your skin

In the U.S. more than 1 million people are diagnosed with skin cancer every year. Incidence has risen rapidly over the past 50 years, and it is now the most common cancer. Increased exposure to sun is a major cause of this rise.

ALL ABOUT SUN

Sunlight is essential for human well-being. Not only does it make us feel good, it also produces heat and illumination, and through plant photosynthesis, the food necessary for our survival. The sun is also our primary source of vitamin D, which is essential for bone health.

Sunlight contains radiation of many different wavelengths, from invisible low-frequency infrared heat radiation, through the visible light spectrum, to invisible ultraviolet rays. Shorter wavelength X-rays also form part of sunlight.

What is UV radiation?

The light rays of ultraviolet (UV) radiation are categorized into three different wavebands called A, B, and C.

The sun is our principal source of UV radiation, although artificial sources can be significant for people such as welders and some hospital workers. Outdoor workers have up to four times the total UV exposure of indoor workers. Although low-intensity fluorescent lights may be a source of UV radiation for indoor workers, this has not yet been proved.

Outdoor activities such as sport and gardening also increase the level of daily UV exposure.

What increases the amount of radiation?

UV radiation is reflected and altered by different surfaces, and damage can be greater under certain circumstances. Exposure increases at high altitude, at low latitude, and closer to the equator. UV rays are strongest during the summer. Reflection of UV rays is increased 25 percent by sand, and 5 percent by water. Reflection is lessened by cloud cover (20–90 percent) and the passage of light through water. It is unaffected by heat, cold, wind, and visible light.

For the last few decades, scientists have been monitoring changes in the ozone layer—the protective layer of the stratosphere. Because of damage caused by human activities, ozone levels have been reduced. This has lead to an increase in the levels of UVB rays reaching the earth.

UVR AND THE SKIN

Two types of UV effect are felt by the skin: acute effects, which appear within a few hours—such as vitamin D production, tanning, or sunburn—or chronic effects, which are cumulative and may not appear for years—such as photoaging or skin cancer. The only nondamaging effect of UV radiation on the skin is the production of vitamin D.

SKIN TYPES

Knowing your skin type is a useful way to predict how your skin will react to the sun. The types below are used by dermatologists to treat skin diseases such as psoriasis with UV light. People with types I to II need to take extra care when deciding how much exposure they can tolerate and how quickly they will respond to treatment.

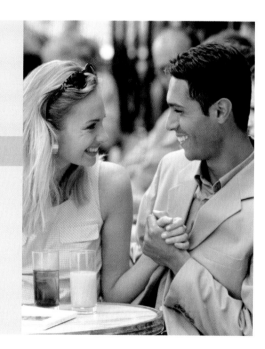

SKIN TYPE	SUN REACTION	TANNING	TYPICAL COMPLEXION
I	always burns	never tans	very fair
II	often burns	tans lightly	fair
III	sometimes burns	tans progressively	fair/medium
IV	rarely burns	tans easily	olive
V	rarely burns	tans deeply	Asian
VI	never burns	tans deeply	Afro-Caribbean

UVA rays pass effortlessly through the ozone layer. They make up the majority of our sun exposure.

Most UVB rays are absorbed by the ozone layer, but enough pass through to cause damage.

UVC rays are the most dangerous but fortunately are blocked by the ozone layer and don't reach the Earth.

VITAMIN D

Vitamin D is formed when UV light converts 7-dehydrocholesterol in the skin into vitamin D_3. A protein in the skin then transports it to the blood and the liver for use.

TANNING

The skin has various mechanisms to protect itself against the harmful effects of the sun.

When the skin is exposed to sunlight, melanin in the epidermis is redistributed toward the surface to absorb the UVA rays. A slight darkening of the skin, called immediate pigment tanning, occurs. However, this is only temporary and fades 3 to 36 hours after exposure.

A second process, called delayed tanning, occurs when the skin is exposed to UVB rays. More melanocytes are produced and melanin production increases, causing the skin to appear darker. The tough outer layer of the skin also thickens to absorb more of the UVB radiation. This two-part process takes one or more days and produces a noticeable tan that can last for weeks or even months.

This thickening and tanning provides some protection against further UV damage but can make the skin more vulnerable to cancer.

WHAT IS SUNBURN?

Sunburn is an inflammatory redness of the skin caused by overexposure to UV radiation, particularly UVB. It is a sign of severe cellular damage. The small blood vessels in the skin dilate and increase the blood flow to the skin's surface, making it red and painful. UVB damage to the DNA of skin cells triggers several inflammatory pathways, causing a swelling of the skin.

A sunburn appears two hours after exposure and develops over the next 24 hours. The skin turns red and blisters, and several days later the dead skin cells peel off. In severe cases, the burn may occur with sunstroke.

IMMUNOSUPPRESSION

UV damage to DNA triggers the release of suppressor T-lymphocytes in the skin. These reduce immune response and subsequently increase the risk of infection or skin cancer.

PHOTOAGING

The damaging effects of UVA can be seen in the premature aging and wrinkling of chronically sun-exposed skin. Collagen and elastin fibers lose

UV intensity

Levels of UV radiation vary depending on the time of day, time of year, altitude, and distance from the equator. UV rays are most intense during midday hours in the summer, although they are always present, even in winter.

their elasticity and appear thickened and clumped. This accounts for the leathery appearance of exposed skin. Photoaged skin also shows epidermal thinning and irregular pigmentation.

SKIN CANCER

UV damages the genes, which can lead to cells losing their normal growth control system. The immune system then fails to identify the abnormal cells, and cancer develops. There are three forms of skin cancer related to sun exposure. Malignant melanoma is linked to sporadic but intense sun exposure, particularly sunburn in childhood. Squamous cell carcinoma and basal cell carcinoma are more treatable and are thought to be linked to more life-long low-grade exposure to UV radiation.

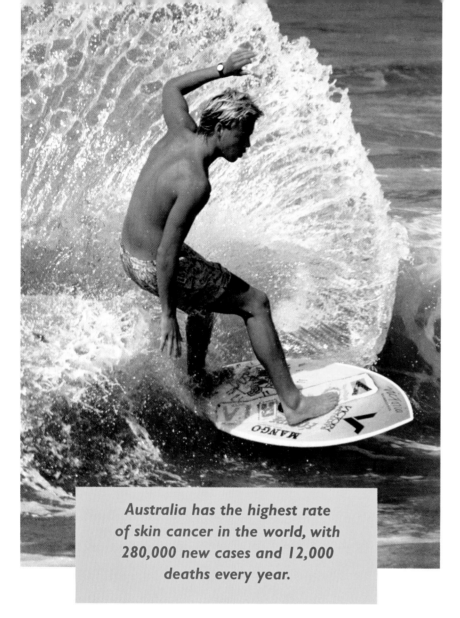

Australia has the highest rate of skin cancer in the world, with 280,000 new cases and 12,000 deaths every year.

grown up with a public health program—known as "Slip, slop, slap"—which advocates

- **Slipping** on a (long-sleeved close-weave) shirt.
- **Slopping** on the sunscreen regularly, especially after swimming.
- **Slapping** on a hat that will cover your neck.

This is sensible advice for everyone.

How sunscreens work

Sunscreens contain organic chemical compounds that absorb UV radiation, and sunblocks contain finely ground particles that reflect UV rays away from the skin. They are available in many forms, including ointments, creams, gels, lotions, sprays, and wax sticks.

All sunscreens are labeled with a sun protection factor (SPF) number that tells you how long you can stay in the sun before you burn. If you would normally burn in 30 minutes, a 15 SPF sunscreen will enable you to prolong that to 15 x 30 minutes. Most recommendations nowadays are that it is not worth using a sunscreen with an SPF of less than 15 or you will be applying it all day.

The factor only applies to UVB radiation, although some manufacturers also attempt to quantify UVA protection. It is also not a good idea to assume that you are safe for hours simply because you are wearing sunscreen: Damage is cumulative, and it is never a good idea to be on a beach during the peak sun hours of noon to 3 P.M. The American Academy of Dermatology recommends never deliberately sunbathing.

If you are going into the sun for more than 20 minutes, you should use a sunscreen. Most people will

WHY DO WE WANT A TAN?

A hundred years ago the idea that a tan could be desirable would have seemed absurd. In countries where most people were fair-skinned, tans were associated with people who worked outdoors and were a badge of low social status.

Attitudes started to change in the 1920s when Coco Chanel introduced the tan as a fashion accessory. At the same time, artificial sun rays began to be used to treat some skin diseases, so being brown came to mean being healthy. After World War II, foreign travel became more desirable and affordable, and a tan was seen as a sign of affluence.

However, even the lightest tan is a sign of skin damage. The rate at which people burn in the sun varies, and this determines skin type. Skin types I and II have fewer melanocytes and tend to burn easily.

Attitudes are now changing as evidence mounts of the damage the sun can do, but many people still seek a "perfect tan." The safest tan is a fake one. There is a wide range of products available to produce a fake tan in a few hours.

SUN PROTECTION

Protection from the sun is extremely important, particularly for children. Since the 1980s, Australians have

EXTRA SUN PRECAUTIONS FOR CHILDREN

Children need special protection from the sun. Even though skin cancer develops mainly in later life, it is sun exposure during childhood that is probably most important in whether we develop it or not.

Severe sunburn before the age of 18 is a risk factor for malignant melanoma: One or more severe, blistering episodes of sunburn in childhood doubles the risk of skin cancer.

Total sun protection
Keep babies out of the sun completely, use high factor sunscreens, and cover them up.

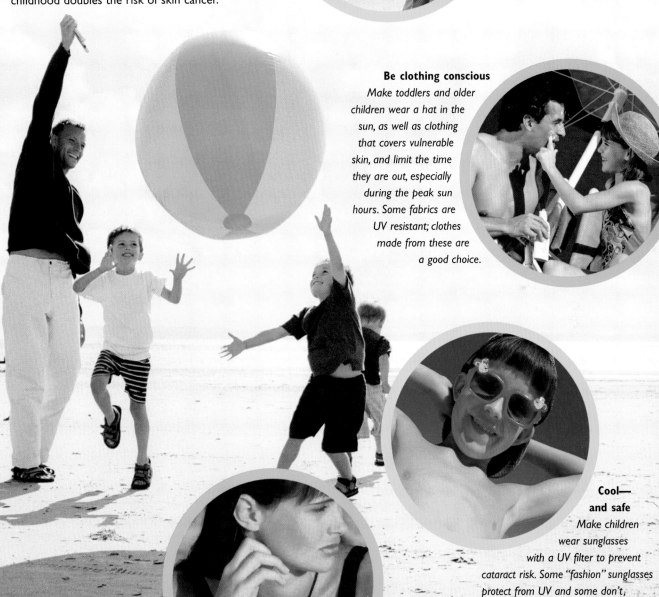

Be clothing conscious
Make toddlers and older children wear a hat in the sun, as well as clothing that covers vulnerable skin, and limit the time they are out, especially during the peak sun hours. Some fabrics are UV resistant; clothes made from these are a good choice.

Cool— and safe
Make children wear sunglasses with a UV filter to prevent cataract risk. Some "fashion" sunglasses protect from UV and some don't, so always check before buying.

Monitor SPF levels
Carry an SPF monitor with a photosensitive strip to tell you how strong the sun is.

VACATIONS AND SKIN PROBLEMS

Preventing skin problems while on vacation is relatively easy as long as you are prepared. Before you go away, check with your pharmacist whether any drugs you are taking might cause a phototoxic reaction in the sun. If they might, cover up and use high SPF sunscreen. Most problems can be treated using the contents of a first aid kit. Rarely, however, they may be more serious, so it is important to watch out for any serious reactions like spasms, shock, or breathing difficulties. If these occur, seek emergency medical help immediately.

USEFUL FIRST AID ITEMS

Vinegar to pour on tentacles to prevent further release of toxins.
Baking soda to make a paste that can help neutralize sting venom.
Antihistamines to ease the itch from bites, stings, or prickly heat.
Acetaminophen for fever or pain.
Witch hazel or aloe vera for burns, bites, and general skin irritations.

Sunburn

Make sure that sun screen is applied for complete cover. If you miss parts of your body, oddly shaped areas of sunburn can appear, on your back or behind your ears, for example. Reapply sunscreen after swimming.

Bites and burrows

Larva nigrans The larvae from dog hookworm are excreted on the sand and can burrow into the skin, leaving a winding track on your legs or buttocks. They move about a tenth of an inch a day. The problem usually resolves spontaneously, but drugs are available to cure the problem.

Sea urchin spines

If you develop painful lumps on your feet after a vacation abroad, you may have unwittingly stepped on a sea urchin spine. These need to be removed with a minor operation before the lesions will settle down. It is good advice, therefore, to wear sandals while swimming.

receive this amount of sun exposure daily, so it is good for your skin to use cosmetics that have daily-use sunscreen in them. Even on a cloudy day, there will be reflected UV light, so use it then as well.

- Sunscreen should be applied to dry skin at least 30 minutes before going outside; use liberal amounts so that it will penetrate the skin and not rub off immediately.
- A high factor sunscreen is ineffective if it washes off during swimming or sweating. "Water-resistant" sunscreen is less effective after 40 minutes in the water and "waterproof" after 80 minutes, so reapply regularly. If you have toweled dry, reapply sooner.
- Lips need cover, so use a sun-protective lip balm with SPF 15 or higher or a sunblock.

Sunscreens are only effective for about two years after manufacture, after which they should be thrown away. The chemicals separate from the solution, so if your sunscreen feels gritty, throw it out.

If you can't remember exactly when the sunscreen was bought, it would be safer to buy a new bottle than to risk inadequate sun protection. In some countries manufacturers are required to put production and use by dates on sunscreens, as for food products.

EMERGENCY TREATMENT FOR SUNBURN

The main symptoms of sunburn are pain and a sensation of heat in the affected skin, which can feel itchy

Insect bites

The severity of the reaction to insect bites varies from individual to individual. Most people get bitten, but not all react. In malarial regions, always be sure to take tablets to prevent malaria, and sleep under a mosquito net.

Sea bather's eruption

Often called "sea lice," this is an itchy rash that comes up in the area covered by the swimsuit and is caused by jellyfish and sea anemone larvae. It can be prevented by showering in fresh water after coming out of the sea.

Stings

Jellyfish stings produce itchy raised red bumps where tentacles touch the skin. If a tentacle is attached to the skin, use tweezers to remove it. *Weaver fish spines* protruding from the sand cause pain and redness when stepped on. Treat by putting the foot in warm water.

We get about 80 percent of our lifetime sun exposure before the age of 20.

Many people use them before a vacation, or have regular "touch-ups" to maintain a tan after a vacation. Yet sunbeds can damage your skin for life.

They are designed to produce a tan by emitting UVA (some have a little UVB). UVA can cause premature aging and also contributes to skin cancer. Tanning beds do not produce the thickening in skin that gradual natural exposure does, so using them before a vacation is not necessarily a protection against burning on vacation. The most important part of the body to protect is the eyes, so always use the mask provided. As little as 30 minutes a week over a period of years may cause increased fragility of the skin.

Tanning beds should not be used by those under 16, by people with skin types I and II (see page 74), by anyone using photosensitive drugs (check the manufacturer's leaflet in the package) or wearing cosmetics (wash before a session), or by anyone who has had skin cancer.

HOW SUN DAMAGES HAIR

Your hair may feel fried after a day at the beach, but hair can't be sunburned because it is not living. Sun exposure damages the hair's natural protective film, because the scalelike cells that cover each individual hair begin to pull off. This will make hair feel fragile, dry, dull,

and tight. The skin may also be red, blistered, or swollen. Some people develop shivering and an elevated temperature; they may also feel very weak. Peeling typically occurs about a week after the episode of burning.

Immediate treatment should include a cool bath for at least 20 minutes, to try to remove some of the excess heat.

Avoiding dehydration is important. If you have been sweating a lot, you may have lost a large amount of body fluid, which must be replaced.

Aftersun creams or 1 percent menthol-in-aqueous cream are soothing for mild sunburn. Acetaminophen can reduce pain and fever, and topical steroids help soothe inflamed skin.

TANNING BEDS

Research suggests that as many as 26 percent of people under 25 have used tanning beds at some time in their lives. The placing of these facilities in health clubs and gyms implies that this is a healthy thing to do, but this is far from the truth.

Why is rain water supposed to be good for washing?

When hard water dries on the skin it feels tight and dry, and this is compounded by the use of detergent-like soaps, bubble baths, and shower gels. Rain water is far softer than tap water in many parts of the U.S., so the deposit left on the skin is reduced, as is the amount of soap necessary to produce lather.

Collecting rain water for bathing is not really practical, so the best compromise is to avoid soap, using soap substitutes for washing, and to moisturize regularly. If you have eczema, it might be a good idea to have a water-softening unit fitted to your washing machine, because the cotton and natural fiber clothing that help with eczema will respond better to washing in softened water. It will also reduce the amount of detergent and fabric softener needed.

ASK THE EXPERT

Wind chill factor
A sea breeze can make temperatures feel deceptively cooler than they really are. Be sure to stay in the shade and avoid the intensity of the midday sun.

and brittle. Hair products are available that contain sunscreen. Hair that has been bleached or dyed is especially prone to sun damage.

SUN AND WIND
The major problems caused to the skin and hair by the wind have to do with its drying effects. The wind makes the ambient temperature seem lower (the chill factor), so it is possible to be fooled into thinking that the sun is not as hot as it really is and not use sufficient protection. When this is combined with the dry air of low humidity, the skin and hair can be damaged far more than necessary.

SWIMMING, THE SKIN, AND THE HAIR
Risks to the skin and hair caused by swimming include
- In the sea: exposure to UV radiation.
- In a pool: chlorine irritation of the skin and eyes, particularly in people who already have eczema.
- Sea and pool: salt and chlorinated water both dry and discolor the hair—chemicals in pool water bind to the hair, which can give it a green or gray tinge. Minerals in

salt water can turn hair a brassy color, especially when combined with sun. Always rinse your hair in fresh water before and after swimming.
- Communal changing rooms can increase the risks of picking up a wart or an athlete's foot infection.

BEAUTY AND THE BEACH
Temporary tattoos are currently fashionable on many beaches worldwide. Although described as henna tattoos, they usually contain other dyes such as PPD (P-phenylenediamine, also known as black henna) and kerosene. These are highly irritant to some skin, and set up irritant contact dermatitis at the site of the tattoo. Postinflammatory hyperpigmentation may occur and the tattoo then becomes semipermanent. Some children have been marked for years by having a black henna tattoo.

The story may not end there, because if you use a hair dye containing the same PPD chemical, you can develop a severe reaction in the scalp. The dye is also used in cheap sandals and can cause a rash on the feet.

Winter and the skin, hair, and nails

Winter is generally safer than summer for the skin, but winter sunlight can still be strong, especially when reflected by snow. Also, certain parts of the body can be affected by alternating extremes of cold and heat.

COVER UP FOR WINTER

Those who engage in skiing and other outdoor activities in snowy climates need proper protection from the cold and also protection from increased exposure to UV radiation. For every 1000 feet in height, UV exposure increases by 5 percent, and snow reflects 80 to 90 percent of UV light, compounding the problem. Layered clothing, consisting of several light, loose layers will trap warm air next to the body and provide adequate ventilation. Thermal underwear is a good choice for anyone who has to spend long periods of time outside in winter, topped by shirt, sweatshirt, jacket, and coat. The layered approach allows you to remove one or more layers indoors when it is warm.

A below-hip-length coat, made from a tightly woven fabric like corduroy, offers the most protection from the cold. A coat with a hood and a warm lining is ideal.

Wear well-insulated gloves to prevent your fingers from freezing. Children (and adults) who play in the snow need waterproof gloves. In extreme conditions, consider wearing mittens over gloves.

Up to 40 percent of total body heat escapes through the head, so it is important to keep it well covered. If you don't have a hood, use a hat, scarf, and earmuffs for added protection. Insulated shoes or boots are a good idea, and in the snow, these must be waterproof. Warm pairs of socks should help prevent chilblains (see this page); if wool socks feel too "itchy," try wearing them over a fine cotton pair. Inside in winter, humidity is reduced because of central heating, so skin can become dry and itchy.

Red cheeks

A ruddy glow on the cheeks is not always a sign of good health. It is often associated with visibly dilated small blood vessels after long, continued exposure to the cold. It is more common in northern regions and is a reflection of the susceptibility of fair-skinned people to cold winds and chilly winters. Applying moisturizer—with sun protection—and petroluem jelly to the cheeks can help.

Chilblains

Chilblains are itchy, burning red swellings that erupt after exposure to cold, but not necessarily freezing, temperatures. Children and the elderly are more commonly affected, but chilblains can occur at any age.

Chilblains are caused by the constriction and expansion of blood vessels in the body's extremities in response to changing temperatures. They usually occur on the toes, heels, fingers, lower legs, nose and ears.

Because there is no effective treatment for chilblains, it is best to try to prevent them: Moisturize your feet, maintain good circulation, and avoid exposure to cold. The itching can be relieved with soothing products such as witch hazel or calamine lotion.

Protect against the elements
Wear well-insulated clothing that allows sweat to escape, but ensure adequate sealing around your wrists, ankles, and neck, where body movement may allow cold air to enter.

SKIING AND SKIN SAFETY

General guidelines on protecting your skin apply while skiing and in other cold weather situations.

- Drink lots of water: The air in winter at high altitudes can be very dry, so it's important to stay well hydrated.
- Don't drink alcohol or caffeine: Alcohol opens blood vessels near the skin's surface, cooling the skin, and both are diuretics, increasing urine production.
- Dress in layers, avoiding cotton: Wet cotton stays wet, but breathable synthetics dry out.
- Take extra clothes for breaks: When you stop skiing, you will need another layer.

- Take plenty of snacks to replenish lost energy: This will help keep you warm and energized.
- Be weather wise: The weather in winter can change suddenly, leading to rapid body chilling. Remember that winter sun is reflected by snow; use skin and eye protection.
- Wear a hat.

Take cover
Dress warmly, but don't forget to protect the skin that is exposed. UV intensity increases with altitude—there is less atmosphere to absorb the sun's rays—so use a high factor sunscreen at all times.

Heat and skin

Persistent exposure to a direct heat source can have a visible effect on the skin. Sitting in front of a fire means that the site of damage is commonly the front of the lower legs. The usual result is a brownish pigmentation in the affected area.

THE DANGERS OF FROSTBITE

Frostbite occurs when body tissues are frozen, which takes only a few seconds in extreme cold. The risk increases in strong winds, at high altitudes, or in touching cold metals. Older people and children are at greater risk than adults, as are those suffering from conditions that reduce the blood supply to the skin, such as diabetes and smoking.

Frostbite generally attacks exposed parts of the body that are at the extremities of the blood circulation, such as the toes, feet, fingers, ears, nose, and cheeks. The condition can be deceptively pain-free, but the affected area appears waxy-white in color until it has thawed. Depending on the length of exposure, deeper structures such as muscles, nerves, arteries, and bone can be affected.

The extent of tissue damage is only appreciated on rewarming. With mild damage, there is redness and pain, and the tissues return to normal in a few hours. More severe damage causes blistering, gangrene, and permanent changes to nerve function, leading to increased sweating and impaired sensation.

Rewarming should be undertaken quickly but gently. The best method is to place the sufferer in a bath at 100°F, for no more than 20 minutes.

GIVING NATURE A HELPING HAND

Most people attempt to improve the skin and hair that nature has given them to some extent—using makeup and hair dyes is the norm rather than the exception. However, more radical methods of modifying appearance are becoming increasingly common in our modern society.

84 *Changing the color, texture, and even length of hair has never been easier with the growing numbers of products for home and salon use.*

88 *The range of makeup products on the shelves is bewildering, but a few carefully selected items will be all that most people need.*

92 *Painting finger and toenails can be a fun way to add a little flamboyance to your life, and extensions can disguise bitten or worn nails.*

94 *Tattooing and body piercing are becoming increasingly popular, but serious thought is vital before the decision is made.*

95 *Cosmetic surgery is not to be undertaken lightly. It is most successful when realistic outcomes are discussed with a reputable surgeon.*

Crowning glories

The condition of our hair has a major impact on how we feel about ourselves and on our self-esteem. There's a lot you can do to enhance your hair if you think it needs it, but professional help and advice is usually recommended.

Of the common chemical applications to the hair, bleaching, dyeing, perming, and straightening all cause damage to some extent, even when carried out by an expert.

STRAIGHT OR CURLY?

Permanent waving, or perming, changes the structure of the hair in order to make the hair shaft produce a desired shape. A lotion penetrates the hair shaft, breaking down its inner structure. The hair then takes the shape of the rod or curler that it is wrapped around. The hair is fixed into this new shape with a neutralizer. Successful perming depends on the manufacturer's formula and also on the expertise of the stylist. The process is a precise one and needs to be carried out correctly in order to ensure as little damage to the hair as possible. If there is too much curl or a lack of curl altogether, dryness and breakage can result.

AFRO-CARIBBEAN HAIR

Afro-Caribbean hair can be woolly, kinky, tightly curled, or wavy. It has a tendency to lack natural moisture and can be very dry. Although it is among the most beautiful types of hair, many who have it feel that it allows little variation, so waving and straightening have become popular. Perming systems can be used to relax naturally curly Afro-Caribbean hair where it tends to be very tight or frizzy. The desired effect is to produce a larger, more controllable curl or wave. Special care must be taken, however, because this type of hair has a tendency to break easily.

There are various temporary methods for straightening Afro-Caribbean hair. The simplest is to set the hair on large rollers when wet, apply stretch or tension, and leave the hair to dry in that position. Hot combs are also used: A metal or alloy comb is heated and repeatedly combed through tight curls. Similarly, electrically heated pressing irons can be used. Care must be taken when applying heat: Follow the manufacturer's advice on timing.

HAIR EXTENSIONS

These are meshes of human or synthetic hair that are attached to existing hair using a special adhesive. They are fitted as close to the roots as possible on small sections of the bottom layers of the hair. The top layer covers the extension points, making them invisible to onlookers.

Wealth of variety
Hair color and texture are genetically determined. Today, however, many treatments are available to modify the hair you were born with if you are not happy with it.

Extensions should be removed after three months, by which time the point of attachment will have moved approximately 1½ inches down the hair shaft as the hair grows. This increases the danger of catching the comb in the adhesive area and ripping the extension—and natural hair—out from the roots. Always choose a professional who has been trained in hair extension work.

If you follow the general guidelines on hair washing (see page 56), using products formulated for extensions, they should need no extra care.

Potential problems
- Hair meshes may be too large, causing strain on the roots.
- Poor-quality adhesives can allow extensions to fall out.
- Too-tight extensions can cause headaches and traction-type loss of the natural hair.
- An allergic reaction to the adhesive may develop.
- Extensions are not wise if you suffer from seborrheic dermatitis.
- Hair extensions may be dislodged by movement against the pillow when sleeping.

COLORING AND BLEACHING
Coloring, or dyeing, and bleaching change hair structure by penetrating the hair shaft. Even semipermanent colors can cause damage to the cuticle of the hair—and semi-permanent and vegetable dyes are not suitable for everyone who wants to dye his or her hair because they do not cover gray hair. They are, however, recommended for hair that has been straightened.

The effects of dyes and bleaches are progressive. If they are left on the hair too long, the outside layer of the

Sales of home dyeing kits in the United States rose rapidly in the 1990s and hit $1.6 billiion in 2001.

hair will weaken and eventually disintegrate, exposing the internal layer of hair. Split ends and fractures then appear in the hair, and it breaks. To keep color-treated hair in good condition, consider the following:
- Start with hair that is in good condition: Before your hair is color treated, have several conditioning treatments.
- Do not wash your hair too often: color-treated hair needs the natural oils produced by the scalp to keep it in optimum condition, so wash your hair only when you need to.

- Use a shampoo and separate conditioner, both designed for color-treated hair.
- Have regular conditioning treatments: Don't wait until your hair is excessively dry before starting to treat it.
- Use a hair dryer on a low setting.
- Have regular trims to keep the ends of the hair in good condition.

COPING WITH BALDNESS
Although usually called male pattern baldness, this condition frequently occurs in women as well. The hormone testosterone is necessary for

Natural hair colorants
Dyes made from the flowers, stems, and barks of plants have been used to color hair for thousands of years. They have a good conditioning effect, but the results can be unpredictable.

Source	Reactions
HENNA	Henna is produced from the powdered leaves of the Egyptian privet Lawsonia. It is commonly used to add red color to the hair.
CHAMOMILE	Chamomile produces a yellow pigment used for brightening the hair; it is still used in some shampoos today. It is not a surface colorant.
INDIGO	Indigo, from the leaves of the indigo plant, gives a blue-black color and, when mixed with henna, produces a variety of colors.
WALNUT	Walnut, from the pod shells of the ripening fruit, produces a yellow-brown color.
QUASSIA	Quassia, from the bark of the quassia tree, was traditionally used with chamomile to brighten the hair. It is still an ingredient of some shampoos.
OTHER SUBSTANCES	Other plant substances—sage, oak bark, cudbear, and logwood—have been used to produce a variety of colors.

this type of hair loss to develop, so it does not occur until after puberty, when both men and women produce testosterone. Some hair follicles are susceptible to testosterone and change from producing fine vellus hairs into stronger thicker terminal hairs. This happens to everyone, but in the condition of androgenetic alopecia, terminal hairs change back and produce vellus hairs again. These hairs eventually stop being produced, and the hair follicles disappear.

There is a typical pattern to the hair loss in men. It begins at the temples with recession of the hairline and progresses to loss over the top of the head. The back and sides of the scalp are not usually affected by this process, even in advanced old age.

In women, the pattern of loss is slightly different: Hair is lost from the temples as in men, but then the hair thins generally over the scalp so that a number of normal hairs are interspersed with the thin hair. This hair loss can speed up after menopause.

The condition is so common that it is difficult to establish whether inheritance plays a part. It does tend to run in families, particularly in women and early onset in men, although the gene(s) involved have not been isolated. It may begin as early as the late teens but generally begins in the late 20s. It is not influenced by environmental factors and can occur in all racial groups.

Psychological effects

The psychological repercussions of losing hair can be enormous both for men and women. The amount of distress is not always proportional to the amount of hair lost or the effect on appearance. It can precipitate a great deal of stress in relationships, and between patient and doctor, partly because no really effective treatment is available.

Because of the enormous distress, people are tempted to clutch at any straw, however expensive, to try to remedy the situation. Physical treatments such as hair implantation, weaving, and hair pieces can disguise the situation, and various treatments are available, two of which—minoxidil and finasteride—have been shown to work in some cases. Both of these drugs were initially developed to treat other conditions but were found to have the effect of stimulating some hair growth as a side effect. The effectiveness of both drugs is variable, but they are worth trying.

It is important to remember that balding is not an illness—nor is it life threatening. In addition, many men in the spotlight periodically shave their heads—and bald men are frequently included in lists of "the world's most attractive men." For those who cannot accept their new appearance, however, the alternatives are to wear a toupee or to have a hair implant.

Wearing a toupee

A toupee is a preshaped base with human or synthetic hair "knotted" into it. This is fixed onto the scalp using a variety of methods.

- **Human hair toupees** tend to lose color after a short while, so they will need regular recoloring. Synthetic hair does not lose its color.
- **Silk-based toupees** are lightweight and allow the scalp to breathe. They can be made from human or synthetic hair and are attached to the scalp using double-sided adhesive tape or spring clips.

- **Polyurethane-based toupees** are lightweight, with human or synthetic hair rooted into a transparent base. When attached to the scalp, the base is invisible and the hair appears to be growing directly out of the scalp. They are fixed in place using either double-sided adhesive tape or liquid glue. Whichever type of toupee you opt for, the base has to fit perfectly, so a template is made of the scalp. Hair samples are taken to ensure a perfect color match, and the density of hair on the toupee will be matched to the density of the hair on the scalp.

Hair transplanting

This involves removing hair from the back of the head to replace hair lost from the front and top areas. Under local anesthetic, a strip of hair-bearing skin is cut from the scalp at the back of the head. The strip is then cut into grafts of up to four hairs, which are inserted into a new area by cutting tiny indentations. During the procedure, which lasts up to five hours, 1,200 to 1,500 grafts may be placed. Depending on the degree of hair loss, three to four procedures, approximately six months apart, may be necessary.

Hair transplanting can successfully reduce the blankness of a balding head. To avoid disappointment, it is important that a patient be informed of the maximum hair density he can expect before getting treatment.

Aging gracefully
Many people adjust quite happily to the onset of gray hair. Men who are able to view progressive hair loss as part of the aging process may come to terms with it more readily than younger men.

A daily makeup routine

There are no "rules" about makeup: Just please yourself. Many people find that makeup enhances how they feel about themselves and some say they feel "naked" without it. But many others are happy not to use makeup on a daily basis.

If your life is a rush from the moment you get up, you might want to keep your daily makeup routine simple and quick or dispense with it altogether. If you have the time and the personality, you might want to do more: Shimmering face powder and glossy lips are too much for some first thing in the morning, but others wouldn't want to leave the house without them.

Now and then, have a good look in the mirror before applying your makeup.

- Are you finding that your usual makeup is just not "working" any more? It may be that your skincare routine could use a change (your skin might have changed because of climate, age, or hormones). Changing to a different moisturizer, for example, might make a difference (see page 53).

- Could your eyebrows be neater? You could consider visiting a salon for a shaping that you can then repeat. If you are going it alone, take it slowly and don't be overzealous.

Remember that makeup works best when it is an enhancement of healthy skin not a substitute for it.

THE SKIN OF THE FACE

Start by cleansing your skin and preparing it with a moisturizer and, if you think you need it, a gel or cream around your eyes. Give your skin a few minutes to absorb this before proceeding, then create a base from a choice of products.

- **Tinted moisturizer** If you have dry skin, apply this on top of your first moisturizer, this can be used instead of a moisturizer. Tinted moisturizer is an excellent timesaver because it's a two in one product and gives a healthy look without covering the skin.

- **Liquid foundation** Apply this with your fingertips (the warmth of your skin will make it glide on more easily) or use latex wedges (readily and cheaply available, so you can throw them out after a few washes). Apply a few dots—you can always add more— to the center of your face and work outward. You might feel that just covering any redness around the nose and the darkness under your eyes is enough.

- **Stick foundation** Apply this to your face straight from the stick and work it in with your fingers or a latex sponge.

- **Cream to powder foundation** Apply this with the (normally included) sponge. This has much more coverage than the other products and is often referred to as a three-in-one product (foundation, concealer, and powder).

Choosing colors

The best color for foundation is a shade that matches your skin tone perfectly—the color should almost disappear. If possible, check this in natural light (take a mirror with you when shopping). For most people a yellow-toned foundation is the most flattering: Pink-toned ones can make white skin look pasty and dark skin look gray. If you have dark skin look for golden tones to bring out the warmth in your complexion.

Working with nature
Often the most successful makeup is unobtrusive: Makeup colors to match natural skin tone, well-shaped brows, and lightly accented lashes can form a good foundation for a flamboyant choice of lip color.

Hiding blemishes

Any blemishes and dark areas can be hidden with concealer. These are available as sticks (use a small brush for more accuracy) and liquid, which comes with its own brush in the bottle or tube.

Find one that is a shade lighter than your skin tone and one that is a match for it. A blemish is less noticeable with a matching covering, and under-eye circles vanish with a shade lighter. Try brands with light reflective particles; they can be extremely effective.

Makeup artists are still divided over applying concealer before or after foundation—experiment to find out which works best for you.

Powder

One thing that makeup artists do agree on is that it is good to "set" your makeup with powder, preferably loose powder applied with a puff. This is because loose particles—as opposed to compact powder which is applied with a flat sponge— "lock" everything in place more easily. The colors that suit most people are yellow-toned or translucent powders. Stay away from the chalky pink ones. Any excess can be brushed away with a big powder brush.

On the other hand, if you're happy with a quick powder of your nose with your compact powder, stick to that. You might, however, want to try loose to see if it makes any difference.

Blush

If you decide to apply blush, opt for the shade that most closely matches your natural flush. Apply it on the apple of your cheek: Smile very widely and aim for the fleshy part, where your natural flush will appear.

Get a proper blush brush if you use a powder blush because the brushes supplied are too narrow and hard. If you use a cream blush, which should be applied with your fingertips, apply it before the "setting" powder.

EYE PRODUCTS

Eye products can have as little or as much impact as you want: You can keep your look minimal, go for glitter eye shadow and false eyelashes, or anything in between.

Start with less of a product: It's always easier to add than it is to take away. Keep in mind that dark colors on the eyes make your lid seem to recede, and light eye colors draw your skin forward.

Shadows

Your basic choices are cream eye shadow, powder eye shadow, and loose eye shadow; all come in a variety of matte, shimmer, sparkle, and gloss versions. Whatever you choose to experiment with, it is usually worthwhile getting some good brushes instead of using the ones supplied with the products; this often makes a product easier to apply and longer lasting.

Pencils and liners

Some people find hard pencils uncomfortable to apply. Liquid eyeliners (either a tube with brush or resembling a felt tip pen) are best kept away from the inner rim of your eyes because they can cause

Baring all
Many women prefer the look of natural skin and do not use makeup regularly. Unadorned skin has natural color.

Subtle difference
The best makeup enhances rather than disguises your natural skin: Colors should be chosen to approximate your natural look.

irritation: Stick to the area below the bottom lashes and above the upper ones. If you want to use eyeliner to define your eyes but find black too harsh for daytime use, you may find that brown, brown-black, or navy blue give a more satisfactory effect.

Eyelash curlers

For an open, awake look, an eyelash curler (metal, plastic, or even heated versions) can work wonders. Makeup artists recommend a simple one that you squeeze over your lashes as close to your eyelid as is comfortable and hold in place for 5 to 10 seconds, repeating if necessary. Be careful when removing it. Only use curlers before applying mascara; otherwise you run the risk of breaking your lashes because they will stick to the curler when you use it.

Mascara

Mascara comes in many colors and varieties, including types that claim to thicken and lengthen the lashes. Whichever you choose, wipe the wand on the tube or with a tissue before applying so you do not overload your lashes. It's easier to apply a second coat than it is to get rid of any excess.

If you want the look of colored lashes but are sensitive to mascara, don't have time to apply it daily, swim regularly, or are a contact lens wearer who finds mascara irritating to the lens, you could consider having your eyelashes tinted; a tint should last 4 to 6 weeks.

LIPS

Some people find the sensation of wearing lipstick unpleasant. If you don't like lipstick but need something to prevent chapping, you could consider a clear lip salve or balm. If you do like lipstick, however, the possibilities are endless: lip-liner, lip-gloss, lip-glaze, and of course lipstick, which is available not just in a stick, but also in tube and jar form.

Some days dabbing on a bit of colored gloss or a hint of lipstick with your fingertips will be enough, but on other days you may want lip-liner, followed by lipstick, and finished off with a high gloss. Whichever you choose, it's worth buying a decent lip brush for applying lipstick. This is especially important when you stray away from neutral tones. You will need a firm, small, flat brush to be able to apply the product accurately; it will also last longer when applied by brush.

Some experts suggest using lip-liner as the first step; others prefer outlining the mouth after the application of lip color. Whichever you find works, remember you don't have to stick to your exact natural lip line. Play around and see what different effects you can achieve by adjusting an arch or a corner.

TRICKS OF THE TRADE

Invest in the best quality makeup and tools you can afford. Good-quality powder and lip brushes, for example, make products easier to apply and will give you a better finish; you'll also find it easier to experiment with styles and colors.

When it comes to selecting products themselves, personal preference, how important makeup is to you, and your budget all play a part. You might, for example, be able to make your favorite, but fairly fast-fading, cheaper foundation last a lot longer if you purchase a better quality setting powder.

Try various brands and price ranges and do not be afraid to experiment. Look at products for different skin types—you may find that you can swap the heavy day cream you've been using for a light moisturizer. Or a skin illuminating makeup base, which you can mix with your regular foundation, might be the answer for those days when you feel that less is more.

Finally, if you find a product or shade you like, don't be discouraged from being loyal because somebody or some magazine tells you it's "out" this season instead of "in." Makeup is all about what you like.

READING LABELS

Many people are allergic to some of the ingredients in everyday cosmetics, especially lanolin used in foundations, powders, makeup removers, and self tanners. Also known as wool alcohol, wool fat, or wool wax, lanolin is produced by the oil glands of sheep. Chemically, it is a wax rather than a fat and contains about 25 to 30 percent water.

If you have been experiencing skin rashes, apply a little of a suspected product to an area of neck, upper arm, or the bend of your arm daily for about a week to see if it causes a reaction. If it does, check labels for lanolin and try to find products that do not contain it.

If you find problems with different products, see if there is an ingredient that pops up on a regular basis and avoid those products for a time to

---

UNDER 8 YEARS

Face paints

Face paints are popular for parties and other special occasions, and most artists will use paints that are safe for children. It's legitimate to ask someone offering face painting in the shopping centre or at a fete what they are using and checking that's is intended for face painting—occasionally craft paints have been used. If you want to buy paints, look for toxic free and easily removable products; those suitable for small children are water based so that they wash off easily. Choose those that are labelled as non-staining, so that if any gets on clothes, it won't mark them. Most shops selling toys or party goods should be able to advise on suitable products.

---

see if that makes a difference. If it doesn't, see your doctor. Your problem might be diet related, for example, or you could be allergic to a substance you hadn't considered.

Skin-lightening products

Skin lighteners are used by many people either to lighten skin overall or to even out patchy pigmentation. Those containing hydroquinone—which can damage skin's genetic material—are legal in the United States but are banned in the European Union. Azelaic acid and glycolic acids have caused skin irritation in some people.

CHILDREN AND MAKEUP

Children have begun experimenting with makeup at younger ages, and in the last few years there has been a trend toward makeup for preteens—cosmetics, skin care, and fragrances

for children who are still in elementary school are now available in shops targeting this age group.

It can be difficult to regulate what preteens buy on shopping trips with friends, but parents have to decide where to draw the line. That doesn't mean that a four year old can't have fun with makeup or that a twelve year old should be discouraged from a lick of moisturizer and a dab of lip gloss in the morning. You can, however, set some guidelines.

- Some schools ban makeup: Support your child's school in this respect.
- Insist that makeup be removed at bedtime.
- Discourage heavy makeup as a "disguise" for blemishes; acne can be treated.
- Draw a distinction between trying out looks with friends at home and what is appropriate, and when, outside the house.

A splash of color

Good-looking nails are often enhanced by a coat of polish, and the range of available colors is such that it is possible to match or complement any outfit. For those who have trouble keeping nails looking good, extensions may be the answer.

NAIL POLISH

Apart from looking good, nail polish protects and strengthens the nails and may help prevent them from splitting and breaking.

Nail polish can be quick and easy to apply (see below). To get the most out of your polish, make sure you apply a good base coat. This will even out any imperfections and soak up any coloring, especially in dark shades of polish that would otherwise stain your nails yellow.

Removing polish

Experts recommend removing polish with acetone-free remover because acetone dries out the skin and nails. Some acetone-free removers have conditioning oils to avoid any damaging nails. Apply it to a cottonball and press it to the nail, giving the remover a few seconds to work its way into the polish and start dissolving it before rubbing.

Nail-biting solutions

Some nail polishes are designed to break nail biters of the habit. These usually consist of polish with an extremely unpleasant taste so that the individual is reluctant to bite. They don't work for everyone (some people put up with the taste) but may be worth trying if you long for longer nails. Hypnosis has also worked for some people.

NAIL TIPS

Since the 1980s, artificial nails, particularly acrylic tips, have become increasingly popular in the United States. They cross gender and occupational barriers: A housewife is as likely as a stressed executive to have them, as is a man who has lost a nail, perhaps through trauma.

A nail extension is a lengthening of the natural nail by either folding a nail form around the fingertip and slightly under the natural free edge or gluing an artificial nail tip on to the tiniest piece of nail bed. Depending on the nail technician and client's preference, any of the following systems can be used to build up the artificial nail:

- Acrylics—sculptured nails with clear or pink and white powder and liquid. These are either air or UV lamp cured (hardened).
- UV gel—a substance like hair gel that is cured under a UV lamp.
- Fiberglass—meshlike fabric strips and resin.
- Silk—silk fabric strips and resin.

Getting nail tips

A nail technician should always start by cleansing both your and his or her hands to avoid passing on germs, bacteria, and infections.

After a basic manicure to clean your nails and to gently push back your cuticles, any skin material attached to your nail bed will be scraped off, the nail bed slightly roughened for better product adhesion, and the free edge shaped. If artificial tips are used, the technician will select the appropriate type and size and will glue them on

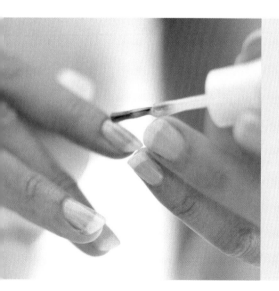

Applying nail polish

To apply polish, divide your nail into three sections, from the cuticle down to the free edge (the tip) and down the left-hand and right-hand sides. Take enough polish onto the brush to cover the whole nail and, avoiding the cuticle, wipe the polish down to the tip. Repeat this on both sides, being careful to avoid the sidewall (the area where your skin touches the nail bed). Finish by wiping the brush around the free edge, so when you look at the nail from the front there is no white edge to be seen. After the first coat has dried, apply a second coat and, for ultimate shine and protection of the new color, a topcoat. Nail polish driers in the form of brush-on liquids, sprays, and little blow dryers are available if you want to speed the drying process.

to your natural nail. They will then be buffed down to be flush with the natural nail. There are many types of tips, including pure white "French" tips (to mimic a French manicure), which do not require buffing.

On a first visit for extensions, it is important not to make them too long: Changing a baby's diaper or using a keyboard might be more difficult than you thought, and you will end up paying the technician a second visit in a few days to have them shortened.

After curing or air drying, the nail extension will be buffed to get an even overall look and correct shape. The extension will be buffed to a sheen, UV gel coated and cured for a gloss effect, or finished off with a clear polish.

A full treatment will take about an hour and a half. "Infill" treatments—in which the gap that appears between the cuticle and the extension as the nail grows is filled in with a nail product and the nail is rebalanced—take about half an hour.

Finding a technician

Most technicians and their clients have heard horror stories of clients' nails being buffed until they bled, leaving people who were willing to put money on the table for a quality service in pain and distress. A self-respecting technician with good training and enough practice before being let loose on real clients should make getting your nails done an enjoyable experience.

The buffing down of tips is important, but the friction created causes pain when a technician buffs the same spot for too long. This is easily avoidable. Also, the lamp used to cure the UV gels becomes hot.

Anybody with sensitive nails will feel this; depending on the person, it might be painful.

As with most things, you get what you pay for. Beware of services that look too cheap—they're probably too good to be true. Nail products are not cheap, and you do pay for an expert's time.

If you take care of extensions (wear rubber gloves when doing chores and do not use them like a new set of garden tools), they can last weeks or months. Regular maintenance treatments will keep any problems, like product lifting, under control and will spot more serious problems like a fungal infection. Experts recommend giving the natural nails a break for a short time every three months or so to prevent the natural nails from weakening.

NAIL ART

Nail art ranges from simple rub-on stencils that are applied over polish to freehand miniature paintings,

Special occasion
Nail artists are coming up with innovative designs all the time, although many can be tricky to do on yourself. The range of available decorative accessories is also increasing.

airbrushed nails, and rhinestones glued to sculptured nails with bold-colored and pastel-colored or glitter acrylic powders. The Internet is a good place to start looking for nail art because many technicians display their art to show their abilities and share their ideas with others.

Fairly simple nail art kits are available in stores, but if you doubt your own artistic talents, talk to your local salon or technician. A salon should be able to show you sample designs and give some idea of prices, which will vary depending on the type of art and the ability of the artist or technician. Some may offer to do one nail for free to give you the opportunity to see if you would like the whole set done.

The American market for toiletries, cosmetics, and perfume is worth about $21 billion and is always growing.

Body art

Human beings of many cultures have been decorating their bodies with paints, inks, and jewelry fashioned from a range of materials for centuries. Body art is increasingly popular in the West, particularly among some groups.

Body art—painting the body or having it tattooed or having one or more areas pierced so that jewelry can be inserted—may be a means for people to establish their individuality or a way of fitting in with a peer group.

BEFORE YOU START
There are several factors involved in making a decision to proceed with a piercing or tattoo.
- Ask yourself why you want to do this. If it is a way to establish individuality, consider other options first: unusual clothes, makeup, or flamboyant jewelry. If you are following the crowd, remember it is your body—you are the person who has to live with your decision, not your friends.

- A recent piercing may close if the jewelry is removed; once the hole is created, this may not happen. The hole should be considered permanent.
- A tattoo should be considered permanent. Although laser treatments have made it is possible to "remove" a tattoo, some inks are more difficult to remove than others, and traces may remain. It is far more expensive—and more painful—to get a tattoo removed than to have one in the first place.

SITE AND DESIGN
Think through where this art is going to be positioned and what sort of designs might be appropriate. Many businesses are still essentially conservative, so multiple piercings or a tattoo in a highly visible place may prejudice a potential employer. It is rarely a good idea to get a tattoo of a partner's name: Relationships break down too often. Tattooists should be able to show you a portfolio; some will create prototypes to your specification, so when you have chosen your artist, discuss possible designs.
- Tongue piercings cause swelling and can take up to three weeks to heal. For a few days, pureed foods may be all a person can tolerate.

Ring the changes
Henna tattoos and other forms of temporary art can be a good alternative to permanent markings and can be changed to suit your mood and circumstances.

Estimates suggest that 50 percent of people who have gotten a tattoo regret it.

- Piercings tend to work best on more static parts of the body, so a navel piercing can be difficult to establish successfully because the area moves so much. Navel piercing can take up to five months to heal.
- Nipple and genital piercings—reputed to increase sexual pleasure—do not appeal to everyone, so although a current partner may be excited by it, a future one may not.
- Tattooing hurts. Generally, areas where there is a lot of muscle, such as the upper arm or thigh, hurt less than those where the bone is close to the surface, like the ankle.
- It takes four weeks for a tattoo to heal; anything that might rub on it should be avoided for another two.
- Tattoos must always be covered by sunblock because the sun can fade them.

GOING AHEAD
Excellent hygiene is vital. Tattooists should use new needles and inks for each client; piercing equipment should also be single use. Talk about possible problems, what to expect during healing, and optimal healing times. Get written follow-up pointers and follow them to the letter.

LAW AND PRACTICE
It is against the law to tattoo anyone under age 18, and no reputable or responsible artist will do so. Some states, such as Oklahoma, have also outlawed body piercing for minors.

Cosmetic surgery

Cosmetic surgery is often confused with plastic surgery. Both types of surgery are performed by trained plastic surgeons, but cosmetic procedures represent an average of only 15 percent of most plastic surgeons' daily workload.

Plastic surgery involves the restoration of form and function to a damaged or malformed body part by reconstructive surgery. The word "plastic" comes from the Greek "plastikos" and Latin "plasticus," meaning to mold or shape. By contrast, cosmetic surgery involves procedures to improve appearance. It is also known as aesthetic surgery. Cosmetic procedures fall broadly into two categories:

- Those that are done to correct a real or perceived physical defect. Procedures that come into this category are breast enlargement or reduction, tummy tucks, tattoo removal, liposuction, correction of ears that stick out, and nose reshaping.

- Those that are done in the pursuit of maintaining a youthful appearance. Procedures such as laser resurfacing, face lift, breast uplift, filler injections, and botulinum toxin injections fit into this category.

Recent research has shown that many patients receive health and psychological benefits from cosmetic surgery. For example, a breast reduction can considerably reduce pain and discomfort and significantly improve quality of life.

A FEW GROUND RULES

Cosmetic surgery differs from most other surgical specialties in that the people who choose to have it are generally not ill and are therefore not really patients at all. They are choosing to have a surgical procedure or cosmetic treatment not because it is going to cure an illness, but because it is going to make them feel better about themselves. Cosmetic surgery is happy surgery—or at least it should be if a few basic rules are followed.

Choose a reputable surgeon

This is easier said than done because medical training and qualifications are frequently difficult for the layperson to understand; and cosmetic surgery, more than any other surgical speciality, is prone to quackery and deceit. The American Society of Plastic Surgeons, established in 1931, is the governing body for surgeons, and the surgeon that you choose for your surgery should be trained in both general and aesthetic surgery. Your surgeon

BODY DYSMORPHIC DISORDER (BDD)

Young adults (20–35) are the most likely age group to suffer from this disorder, which is equally prevalent among men and women. It is characterized by preoccupation with a nonexistent or minimal cosmetic defect (nose, cleft chin, blemish, breast size) and a persistence in seeking medical attention to fix it surgically.

How do sufferers behave?

- Constantly checking him or herself in the mirror.
- Constantly seeking reassurance about the defect from others.
- Always taking great pains to disguise or hide the perceived defect.
- Withdrawal from social meetings and work.
- May be clinically depressed—sometimes suicidal.
- May have other obsessive traits.
- May have a dependent, anxious, or fearful personality.

How is it treated?

- NOT by surgery.
- Cognitive behavior therapy can be effective.
- Pharmacotherapy—mainly by the use of serotonin reuptake inhibitors (SRIs) that are used to treat depression, obsessive–compulsive disorder (OCD), and other anxiety conditions.

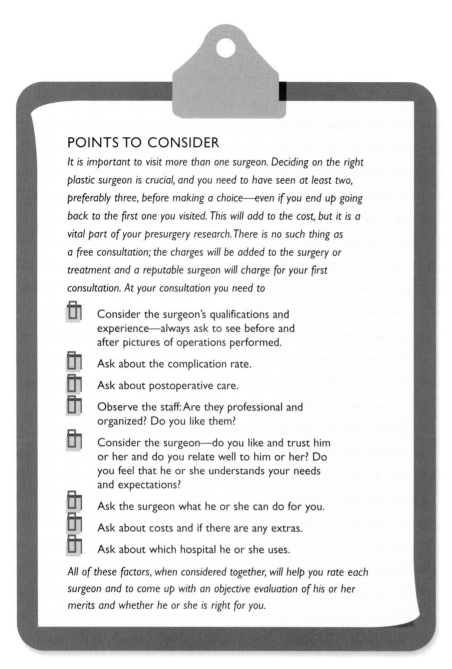

POINTS TO CONSIDER

It is important to visit more than one surgeon. Deciding on the right plastic surgeon is crucial, and you need to have seen at least two, preferably three, before making a choice—even if you end up going back to the first one you visited. This will add to the cost, but it is a vital part of your presurgery research. There is no such thing as a free consultation; the charges will be added to the surgery or treatment and a reputable surgeon will charge for your first consultation. At your consultation you need to

- Consider the surgeon's qualifications and experience—always ask to see before and after pictures of operations performed.

- Ask about the complication rate.

- Ask about postoperative care.

- Observe the staff: Are they professional and organized? Do you like them?

- Consider the surgeon—do you like and trust him or her and do you relate well to him or her? Do you feel that he or she understands your needs and expectations?

- Ask the surgeon what he or she can do for you.

- Ask about costs and if there are any extras.

- Ask about which hospital he or she uses.

All of these factors, when considered together, will help you rate each surgeon and to come up with an objective evaluation of his or her merits and whether he or she is right for you.

should also be board-certified. Look for the ASPS logo when selecting a platic surgeon. This shows that the surgeon is certified by the American Board of Plastic Surgery or by the Royal College of Physicians and Surgeons of Canada. Membership in ASPS is voluntary, so most reputable surgeons will belong.

Qualifications are not a guarantee of excellence, but they have a good place to start. Your psysician can recommend a reputable surgeon, but

many people are reluctant to consult a physician about cosmetic concerns. You can also try the ASPS website, www.plasticsurgery.org.

One factor that may set a reputable surgeon apart is a decision not to operate. Trained and experienced surgeons will refuse to operate when they believe that the requested surgery is not required or is inappropriate. They may refuse to operate if they have reason to believe that the request for surgery comes from

someone other than the patient (for example, a boyfriend offering to pay for breast enlargement surgery). They are also trained to identify patients with a psychological disorder for whom surgery would not be the best treatment. Examples of this are people suffering with body dysmorphic disorder or those who are depressed and who believe that a facelift will find them a man or get them a new job. In these cases, the reputable surgeon may suggest a psychological assessment before surgery and may ultimately exercise the right to refuse to operate.

Seek counseling

Counseling is essential. You must discuss surgery with someone who can be objective. Your physician may be your first port of call, or you may wish to discuss your ideas with a close friend or relative. There are professional beauty counselors who will advise on the best surgeon for the procedure you want and who will provide information about the procedure and postoperative care. Make sure that these counselors are independent; they should charge for consultations. Beware of counselors offering free consultations or those attached to cosmetic surgery clinics: They may be salespersons in disguise. Their bottom line is making money, and they may not have your best interests at heart. *Never* consent to surgery without first having seen your surgeon on at least one, preferably two, occasions.

Know your budget

This is very important, and people frequently fall prey to questionable deals because they use cost as the major determinant for their choice of surgeon and hospital. In a good cosmetic surgery practice, the patient coordinator or receptionist will deal with money issues; the surgeon will not get involved. Get an idea of the costs involved when calling for an appointment. If the costs for a facelift are out of your range, say so. The surgeon might be able to help you achieve your objective by performing a reduction of the bags under your eyes or laser resurfacing while you save for the facelift. It is worth waiting an extra year to have surgery done by a qualified, experienced surgeon. Surgeons who are prepared to do deals will cut costs somewhere, and it will not be on their profits. The cost—not only financial—of repairing the damage done by an inexperienced or unqualified surgeon can far outweigh the cost of the surgery.

Be realistic about outcomes

Again this is difficult, and good surgeons will not operate if they feel that a patient's expectations are unrealistic and unachievable. There is no point in taking a photograph of Jennifer Lopez to your surgeon and asking for eyes like hers if you are a 50-something sun worshipper who has smoked for years. A photograph of how you looked ten years ago, for example, will give something more realistic to aim for.

Some surgeons use computer technology to "morph" a digital picture of your face or body so that you can see how you will look after surgery. The technique can be helpful, but remember that surgery is not a precise science and the result might be different from what you were shown. Also beware of this technique if it is used as a sales exercise because the results cannot be guaranteed.

COMMON PROCEDURES

Nonsurgical procedures include
- injections of botulinum toxin;
- injections of "fillers" such as collagen to plump out fine lines and wrinkles, raising them to the level of the surrounding skin;
- chemical peels (see page 124);
- dermabrasion and laser therapy for wrinkles, scars, tattoos, or birthmarks (see pages 125–27).

Not all nonsurgical procedures are exclusively in the domain of plastic surgeons: Some dermatologists also perform them.

BOTULINUM TOXINS

Injection of botulinum toxins is the most popular nonsurgical cosmetic procedure in use today. It is becoming a "lunchtime" procedure: It takes only minutes and involves no anesthetic or sedative. The rapid increase in its use—500 percent in the last year—is mainly because the Food and Drug Administration (FDA) approved Botox® (Allergan Inc.) for cosmetic use. Botox® is not the only botulinum toxin available, but its name has become synonymous with the treatment. Dysport® (Ipsen) and NeuroBloc® (Elan Pharma) are also available in the UK and the United States.

None of these products is licensed for cosmetic use in the UK (although this situation may change): These are prescription-only medicines, and you need to be very careful whom you choose to administer them. Ideally, a qualified medical practitioner

should give them, and at the very least, if they are to be given by a nurse, a doctor must have seen you prior to writing the prescription.

How do botulinum toxins work?

Botulinum toxins are given as injections into the muscles that underlie frowns, furrows, and lines—mainly the frown lines, crow's feet around the eyes, and horizontal forehead lines. Botulinum toxin is a neurotoxin that works by relaxing the muscles and preventing them from contracting. Because the muscles are unable to contract, the lines above them disappear. If the lines or furrows are very deep, it is sometimes necessary to "fill" them with an injectable filler such as collagen after the botulinum toxin treatment has had time to take effect.

Botulinum toxins take two days to two weeks to reach their maximum effect. The injections need to be repeated after three to six months.

Side effects of botulinum toxins

It is possible to have an allergic reaction to the toxin when injected, although this is extremely rare and is probably caused by the albumin solution in which it is suspended. After a period of repeated injections, some people develop antibodies to the toxins, which are then unable to achieve the desired effect.

Poor placement of the injections can lead to drooping of the features, particularly if the injections for

Nonsurgical procedures are the most common cosmetic interventions performed by cosmetic surgeons and are most frequently performed on people under age 50.

forehead lines are given too far from the center: This can cause the eyelids to droop. This is only temporary but may nevertheless cause distress.

FACELIFTS

When most people think of cosmetic surgery, the image that comes to mind is of facelifts and of the taut, often overstretched look that seem to typify the operation. The technical term for a facelift is rhytidectomy—literally, removal of lines. The operation appeals mainly to women from their mid to late 40s up to the late 60s, but there is some evidence that women as young as 30 are considering this surgery, and men are increasingly requesting it, too.

Types of facelift

There are four basic types of facelifts—if the surgeon you consult only does one type, consult someone else. All faces differ in the degree and extent of aging, as well as in the sites of aging: A good surgeon will recognize and advise the best technique for an individual face. There is no such thing as a formula facelift.

The most popular technique is the SMAS (submuscular aponeurotic system) lift, in which excess skin is removed and the remaining skin is redraped optimally. It also includes tightening the SMAS layer (underlying muscles), and excess fat under the chin may be removed by liposuction.

Some surgeons may perform an extended SMAS lift. This procedure is the same as the SMAS lift except that more tension is placed on the layer of muscles rather than on the skin.

The subperiosteal or MASK lift can be performed with an endoscope. The procedure involves freeing the

Facelift markers
Prior to surgery, sterile, colored marking pens are used to indicate incision lines and geographical reference points on the skin.

muscle from the bone so that it can be tightened and so that excess skin can be pulled up and excised.

The most extensive technique is a composite facelift, which involves removing skin from the upper and lower eyelids, a brow lift, and tightening of the face and neck muscles. Only very experienced surgeons are capable of performing this technique.

Getting the facts

It is not necessary to know all the technical details, but if you are considering a facelift you should know enough to be able to question your potential surgeon wisely. You should be aware that all facelifts involve making an incision at the temple (in the hairline) and that the different techniques create incisions—and hence scars—at other places, mainly around the ears.

A facelift is major surgery—it will take three hours minimum under a general anesthetic. The recovery time, for those who obey the postoperative instructions to the

letter, is a minimum of two weeks before feeling comfortable in public again, and it can be several months before all of the scarring and swelling finally settle down into the finished result. It is also important to remember that a facelift will not last forever. It will probably need to be repeated after about ten years.

EYELID SURGERY

Eyelid surgery (blepharoplasty) is performed on adults of all ages for two main reasons: to correct signs or effects of aging or to correct inherited traits. In the latter case, people may seek surgery as early as their 20s or 30s.

Reasons for seeking eyelid surgery

- Loose skin hanging down from the upper eyelids can obscure vision.
- Excess skin can obscure the natural fold of the upper eyelids.
- Droopiness of the lower eyelid shows the white below the iris.
- Bags and dark circles with or without excess skin and fine creepy wrinkles of the lower eyelid appear.
- A puffy appearance of the upper eyelids—people may say your eyes look tired.

Eyelid surgery itself generally involves the removal of excess skin and fatty tissue from the upper or lower lids or both. The incisions can usually follow the natural contours of the eye and are well camouflaged when healed. Many surgeons are using a new approach called a transconjunctival incision. This results in no visible scars at all as the incisions are made inside the eye.

Complications include the risk of hematoma formation—an accumulation of blood under the skin that may require removal. The eyes may also become dry, increasing the risk of infection. It usually takes at least two weeks for all bruising to subside, and the result may take two or three months to become apparent.

Blepharoplasty is not the answer to all eye area problems: Sagging eyebrows may be best treated by a brow or forehead lift, for example, and crow's feet may be smoothed by laser resurfacing or a chemical peel.

BREAST AUGMENTATION

Breast augmentation or enlargement is very popular, particularly in women who have completed their families and who would like to put some shape back into their breasts.

There are many types of implants available, and your surgeon will discuss the most appropriate type for you. You need to be realistic when choosing your new size. Reputable surgeons will not increase a woman's bra size by more than two sizes at any one time. This is because the skin would have to stretch too much, which could be uncomfortable and increase the risk of capsule formation.

Breast implants are placed on top of or underneath the breast muscle, through an incision on the side of the breast. There will be a scar that may be visible when it has healed.

Following surgery under a general anesthetic, you will be tightly bandaged for about a week. After this time, the surgeon will see you again to remove the stitches. You must wear a supportive bra (like a sports bra) for several weeks following the surgery to ensure that the implants fix in the right place.

Complications of breast augmentation surgery are infection, hematoma formation, and the formation of a capsule around the implant. This is a normal healing process, but sometimes it occurs excessively and the capsule may contract and compress the implant, causing the breast to feel harder than normal and perhaps distorting its shape. Occasionally, implants need to be removed or replaced because of these complications.

BREAST REDUCTION

Breast reduction surgery is sought by women who feel that their breasts are too large or whose breasts are so large that they produce symptoms such as back and shoulder pain and also psychological distress. This is major surgery performed under a general anesthetic, so you need to be fit and well before being considered for it.

The most common method of reducing the breasts involves three incisions. One incision is made around the areola. Another runs vertically from the bottom edge of the areola to the crease underneath the breast. The third incision follows the natural curve of the breast crease. After excess breast tissue, fat, and skin have been removed, the nipple and areola are shifted to a higher position. The areola, which in large breasts has usually been stretched, is also reduced in size. Skin that was formerly located above the nipple is brought down and together to reshape the breast. Liposuction may be used to improve the contour under the arm. Usually, the nipples and areolas remain attached to underlying mounds of tissue, and this allows for the preservation of sensation. The ability to breastfeed may also be preserved, although this cannot be guaranteed.

Complications include bleeding, infection, and poor healing. Occasionally, the breasts appear uneven in shape or size and sensation in the nipples is reduced or absent. Minor changes may be made at a later date if required.

LIPOSUCTION

Liposuction is the single most common cosmetic surgery procedure for both men and women. People seek it at all ages, usually for isolated pockets of fat in the buttocks, thighs, tummy, upper arms, or chin. The best results are obtained when the skin has enough elasticity to spring back, so that a smooth and unwrinkled outline is achieved. Liposuction should not be used as a substitute for weight loss, and reputable surgeons recommend that patients are at their desired weight before undergoing the procedure.

Fat is removed by inserting a small hollow tube (a cannula) through one or more tiny incisions near the area to be suctioned. The cannula is attached to a vacuum pressure unit by tubing and is guided by the surgeon; the suction device literally sucks away unwanted fat.

Following surgery, the areas that have been treated will be bruised and there may be some swelling. The surgeon will apply tight pressure dressings or garments to help produce a smooth, even contour; these must be worn for as long as instructed. There may be some numbness in the treated areas, but feeling will return after two to three weeks as the bruising and swelling subside.

The results of liposuction are permanent provided that your postoperative weight is maintained. If you do gain weight, it may be better distributed than previously.

3

What happens when things go wrong

Knowing what can go wrong

The skin's large surface area and complex makeup make it vulnerable to a wide variety of ailments—some inherited, some the result of infection, and some brought about by contact with the environment.

AGE-RELATED PROBLEMS

Some skin problems are more common at one age than at another. For example, a child is more vulnerable to infection, whereas an aging adult bears the effects of many years of exposure to ultraviolet radiation.

Growing up

A baby's skin is more vulnerable than that of an adult, and therefore contact with the environment is the cause of most skin problems at this age. Infantile eczema, for example, is thought to be provoked by environmental

MORE COMMON

ACNE	ECZEMA
Almost 100 percent of people between 12 and 17 years old have at least an occasional blemish. More than 40 percent of cases are severe enough to require treatment by a doctor. Acne is most common in teens but can strike at any age.	About 15 million people in the United States have some form of eczema, including 10 to 20 percent of babies. In about half of these babies, the condition will largely clear up between the ages of 5 and 15. This condition usually appears during infancy.

factors. Infections that affect the skin (caused by bacteria, viruses, or fungi) are common. The traditional childhood illnesses chicken pox (see page 137), measles, and German measles (rubella) produce skin rashes, and are all caused by viruses. Because the immune system is less well-developed than it will later become, infections such as impetigo, a bacterial skin infection (see page 143), may persist or recur throughout childhood. Warts (see page 155) are another common skin infection, in this case caused by a virus.

Problems on all fronts
Skin faces daily assault from many sources, so skin problems are common. However, many are easy to avoid or treat.

sun and wind damage

aging

infections

cleanser damage

trauma

It is important to protect a child from too much ultraviolet (UV) radiation from sunlight. This is because exposure to excessive amounts of UV radiation in childhood is thought to be a major cause of skin cancer in later life, especially if a child suffers sunburn: A single episode of blistering sunburn can be enough to trigger a cancerous growth.

Acne (see page 134) is the main skin problem for teenagers, and it may persist into the 30s and even beyond.

Getting older

As we age, the effect of UV radiation takes its toll, with creases, lines, and wrinkles becoming common on areas of the skin exposed to sunlight. As damage from UV rays accumulates, so does the risk of skin cancer. In addition, cigarette smoking promotes premature aging of the skin that is especially noticeable on the face. Detergents such as dish-washing liquid will take their toll on the condition of hands and nails unless protective gloves are worn.

What do liver spots have to do with the liver?

The answer is nothing, although they were once believed to be a sign of liver malfunction. A liver spot (also known as a sun spot or age spot) is called a lentigo by the experts (the plural is lentigines or lentigos). They are flat, harmless brown discolorations of the skin found on sun-exposed sites of the body such as the face, neck, and backs of the hands. They are caused by long-term sun exposure and can only be prevented by avoiding the sun before age 40. The new treatment for them is alpha- and betahydroxy acid gels and peels. A liver spot on the face may occasionally develop into a slow-growing malignant melanoma, so if you notice a liver spot changing, get a referral to a skin specialist.

ASK THE EXPERT

LESS COMMON

FOOT INFECTION
About 5 percent of the U.S. population has foot infections, including athlete's foot, other fungal infections, and warts every year.

PSORIASIS
Psoriasis affects more than 7 million Americans, about 2.6 percent of the population. More than 150,000 new cases are reported every year, 20,000 of them in children under 10. It is most commonly diagnosed between ages 15 and 35.

VITILIGO
About 1 to 2 percent of the world's population, 40 to 50 million people, suffer from vitiligo, 2 to 5 million in the U.S. It generally develops before age 40 and affects all races and genders equally.

SKIN CANCER
Most skin cancer is non-melanoma cancer, such as basal or squamous cell carcinoma. More than 1 million of these cases are diagnosed every year. About 54,000 melanomas are diagnosed every year, causing 7,500 deaths. About 2,000 die from non-melanoma skin cancer. Skin cancer is the most common cancer.

LUPUS
About 1.5 million Americans have a form of lupus. Lupus is much more prevalent among people of color, and 90 percent of cases occur in women. Systemic lupus usually develops between ages 15 and 45.

GENETIC INHERITANCE

Some skin disorders have a genetic cause. The common conditions eczema and psoriasis fall into this category, but it is thought in both these cases that environmental factors may also be involved. If there is a history of a severe inherited skin disorder in the family, a skin biopsy can be taken from a fetus, making prenatal diagnosis of rare conditions such as epidermolysis bullosa, ichthyosis (see page 143), and albinism (see page 135) possible.

GEOGRAPHIC AND RACIAL FACTORS

Skin diseases vary in frequency from one part of the world to another. This can often be because a particular infectious disease is more prevalent in a particular part of the world, as with leprosy (see page 145). In addition, the varying amount of pigment in the skin and the differing nature of the hair follicles in different racial groups make those groups more or less prone to certain problems with skin, nails, and hair: Skin cancer, for example, is far more common in Caucasians than in people of African origin.

CLIMATE AND THE WEATHER

Our skin protects us from the weather, but in the process it is inevitably changed—often not for the better. These changes are mainly brought about by exposure to UV rays—the sun is the biggest influence on the skin's health and appearance. Wind, rain, and snow, however, can all influence the feel and look of the skin and hair, making skin too dry, rough, or sore. Lips are particularly prone to chapping in cold weather. Chilblains (see page 137) can develop on exposed hands and feet in very cold weather.

ECZEMA (DERMATITIS)

Eczema and dermatitis (see page 138) are often thought
to be separate conditions, but as far as dermatologists are
concerned, the words are interchangeable. The primary
defect in eczema is a breakdown in the barrier function
of the skin, allowing antigens such as dust mites and
bacteria to penetrate the skin. This barrier defect may
be inherited (atopic eczema often runs in families and
is associated with asthma, hay fever, and urticaria) or
triggered by an allergic response to a particular substance
or by long-term exposure to some kind of irritant such as
a detergent. Allergic contact dermatitis is most often set
off by contact with nickel, but chemicals in glues, dyes,
leathers, skin creams, or cosmetics are all common causes.

SKIN TUMORS

There are many types of cells in the epidermis and dermis
that can undergo changes from disease processes, and
each cell type develops its own form of tumor. For
example, basal cells in the epidermis can proliferate to
produce harmless seborrheic keratoses or develop into
malignant basal cell carcinomas. Melanocytes can
produce harmless pigmented nevi (moles) or malignant
melanomas that can be fatal if not diagnosed early (see
page 130). The skin may also be the site of secondary
spread of cancers that first developed in other parts of the
body, such as the breast or the lymphatic system.

FUNGAL INFECTIONS

Skin-loving fungi called dermatophytes feed on keratin
and cause various problems, including athlete's foot (tinea
pedis), toenail infections (onychomycosis), ringworm of

In the United States, 53,600 new cases of malignant melanoma are diagnosed every year, and 7400 people die from the disease.

the body (tinea corporis), and scalp ringworm (tinea
capitis). Fungi that affect humans can come from humans,
animals, or soil; the inflammatory response is most severe
with fungi from soil, less severe with animal sources, and
milder when the source is human.

TRAUMA

The skin has amazing healing properties and is able
to restructure itself even after major injury. However,
sometimes scar tissue does not stop forming but
continues to grow at the site of injury. Excessive growth
of connective tissue beyond the original trauma site is
referred to as a keloid (see page 144). Keloids are most
common on darker skins and on the head and neck.

NUTRITIONAL DEFICIENCIES

A poor diet will often affect the skin. In regions where
famine is common, the disease kwashiorkor, caused by
malnutrition, leads to darker skin and the development of
red-brown hair. Iron deficiency can make nails brittle and
spoon-shaped and may also cause hair to thin. There is an
association between pernicious anemia (an autoimmune
disorder that prevents absorption of vitamin B_{12} in the
stomach) and gray hair and blue eyes. (Premature graying
of the hair is thought to be an independent autoimmune
disorder.) Deficiencies of calcium can cause brittle nails,
lack of copper can cause hair loss, and not enough fatty
acids can lead to dry skin and hair. A deficiency of niacin
may cause dermatitis, lack of vitamin B_6 can cause acne
and hair loss, and anyone lacking in vitamin A can suffer
from acne, dry hair, and thicker, rougher skin.

HAIR LOSS

Hair loss can be caused by genetic factors (male pattern
baldness); it can also result from drug treatment for some
other illness (it is a common side effect of chemotherapy),
from stress, or from a medical disorder (see page 141).

A typical case of eczema (dermatitis) on an arm
*The inflamed itchy skin that characterizes eczema/dermatitis
affects one in five of all patients who visit a dermatologist's office.
These patients may be any age.*

Who's who—skin, hair, and nail specialists

Experts in diseases and disorders of the skin, hair, and nails tackle a wide range of problems, from the minor—removing a benign cyst, for instance—to major life-threatening conditions such as skin cancer.

PRIMARY CARE PHYSICIAN

The family doctor is most people's first port of call with a problem with the skin, hair, or nails. Many physicians have specific experience in dermatology, either from working in a hospital clinic under the supervision of a dermatology team or from extra study and gaining diploma qualifications.

PLASTIC SURGEON

A plastic surgeon is a doctor who first trained in general surgery and then undertook further training in plastic and reconstructive surgery. Plastic surgery aims to restore parts of the body that are deformed or damaged; the cause may be congenital, an injury of some kind, or the result of surgery for another problem.

ONCOLOGIST

An oncologist investigates and treats cancer. In cases of cancer of the skin, it is common for an oncologist and a dermatologist to see the patient together in order to work out the best possible treatment. This may involve the use of drugs, surgery, radiation, or a mixture of these.

OTHER HOSPITAL SPECIALISTS

All the following doctors are also hospital-based specialists, who in the course of their work become involved in the diagnosis and treatment of many different diseases and disorders of the skin.

- A radiologist uses imaging techniques such as X-rays, ultrasound, MRIs, and CT scanning to investigate various skin problems.
- A radiologist employs X-ray and radioactive substance therapies to treat cancers of the skin.
- An immunologist, based in the laboratory, investigates illness using techniques based on the workings of the body's immune system.
- An immunotherapist treats skin diseases, often skin cancer, with immune proteins to prevent the tumor cells from growing and dividing.

DERMATOLOGIST

This is a doctor who has specialized in diagnosing and treating disorders of the skin, hair, and nails. Most dermatologists have their own special subjects and research interests, and many have a great deal of experience in skin surgery and laser treatment. The majority have a lot of expertise in all dermatology problems as well as their own special interests. They work closely with oncologists, plastic surgeons, and other medical specialists.

- A histopathologist is a laboratory-based pathologist who specializes in the analysis of body tissue samples.
- A microbiologist tests blood, urine, and body tissues for microorganisms that may be the cause of an abnormality in the skin, hair, or nails.

TRICHOLOGIST

Trichologists are specialists in the diagnosis and treatment of hair disorders such as hair loss. They are generally nonmedical experts (whose treatments have not always been subject to rigorous medical testing). Some dermatologists have a special interest in hair disorders.

PODIATRIST

Podiatrists specialize in disorders of foot function such as flat feet or overlapping toes and may supply shoe inserts to correct problems and protect problem areas. They also treat foot and nail problems such as corns, bunions, and ingrown toenails. In some countries, doctors who treat these problems are specialists called chiropodists. The distinction between the two specialties is not usually made in the United States.

FINDING OUT WHAT IS WRONG

Because they are highly visible, skin problems can be among the easiest medical problems to diagnose. However, because several conditions produce similar-looking lesions, doctors can also call upon a battery of tests to identify the exact problem. These include blood tests, laboratory analysis of a sample of the rash, allergy testing, and the use of dyes to track the spread of cancer.

Medical history and examination

Dermatology differs from other branches of medicine in that the problem is usually clearly visible. Keen eyes, a bright light, and possibly a magnifying glass are often all that is necessary for a doctor to make a diagnosis.

WHAT THE DOCTOR LOOKS FOR

The doctor will want to know when the problem started, where on the skin it originated, how it seemed to spread, and all details of any symptoms such as itching, pain, burning, blistering, or fever. What seems to aggravate symptoms? Details of any methods the patient has found to alleviate symptoms are also very useful.

The doctor will ask the patient for a full description of any past skin problems and their treatment, and will also want a general medical history, including details of all previous illnesses. Do any members of the patient's family have any skin troubles now (indicating the possibility of a transmissible infection) or have they had any in the past (indicating the condition might be inherited)?

The doctor will want a full list of any medications being taken by the patient. Many drugs can have an effect on the skin either directly, as with an allergic reaction, or by altering the way the body reacts to sunlight. Details of the patient's diet are also asked for.

Information about the patient's job is important. What chemicals does the patient come into contact with? Do symptoms worsen at work? Hobbies must also be taken into account. Gardeners, for example, can develop allergic rashes brought on by contact with certain plants. Tropical fish can pass on a skin infection that would be very difficult for a doctor to diagnose without knowing that the patient keeps a fish tank. Has the patient been on vacation recently? Tropical worms, coral, and sea urchins can all leave their marks on the skin.

THE EXAMINATION

To examine the skin properly, the lighting should be good. Most doctors prefer bright daylight. The doctor often needs to inspect the entire surface of the skin; it is always possible that some lesions may not have been noticed by the patient. If the face is affected, it helps the doctor if a patient does not wear makeup.

Describing changes in moles

Any pigmented mole, whether new or old, that shows three or more of the seven listed features, especially one of the first three, will be regarded as suspicious by a doctor and will need to be removed and examined under a microscope.

- *Is an existing mole getting larger or starting to grow vertically? If a patient is over the age of 40 or so, is this a new mole growing?*

- *Does the mole have an irregular outline?*

- *Are there various shades of color in the mole rather than it being all one color? Any black coloration is particularly suspect.*

- *Is the mole greater than .24 in. in diameter?*

- *Is the mole inflamed or has it developed a reddish edge?*

- *Is the mole crusting, bleeding, or oozing?*

- *Does the mole itch or hurt?*

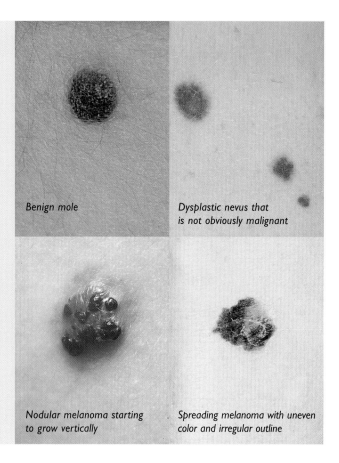

Benign mole

Dysplastic nevus that is not obviously malignant

Nodular melanoma starting to grow vertically

Spreading melanoma with uneven color and irregular outline

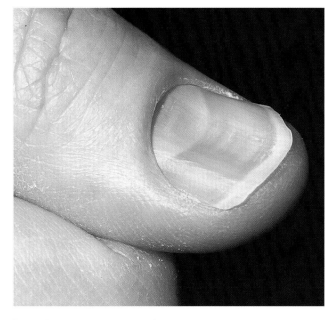

The nail condition koilonychia

The development of thin, brittle, concave, "spoon-shaped" nails can occur as a result of anemia caused by iron deficiency. Why anemia causes the nails to take this shape is not known. If the anemia is treated, the nails should return to their normal condition and shape.

THE SKIN AND NAILS AS BAROMETERS OF HEALTH IN GENERAL

There are a lot of diseases and disorders that affect the skin, hair, or nails in addition to other organs in the body. A patient with a skin problem of some kind may be surprised to learn, for example, that the problem is in fact diabetes or a liver or respiratory disease.

Symptoms of the skin, hair, and nails that indicate disease elsewhere in the body include

- **Finger clubbing** This is a swelling of the soft tissues of the ends of the fingers, which makes the nails appear swollen and more rounded. It is a sign of lung and heart disease.

- **Liver palms** Redness of the palms may occur in pregnancy, but it is usually associated with liver disorders.

- **Facial hair** Increased facial hair in women can be a pointer to an underlying hormonal imbalance such as that found in polycystic ovarian syndrome.

- **Koilonychia** This is a spooning and thinning of the nail plate and is often associated with iron deficiency.

- **Beau's lines** These are horizontal lines that appear in the nails shortly after an illness such as a chest infection.

Tests and investigations

Although many skin problems are immediately obvious to the trained eye and easy to diagnose, some can be more difficult to identify accurately. Physicians and hospital clinics can carry out an array of tests to help them to reach a diagnosis.

TESTS PERFORMED BY THE DOCTOR

After listening to a patient's story and carrying out a close physical examination, a family doctor may undertake further tests.

Blood tests

Sometimes a skin problem is an external sign of an internal illness such as liver disease or a cancerous tumor or of a vitamin or mineral deficiency. For example, dry skin accompanied by hair loss might indicate an underactive thyroid gland; jaundice and spider nevi (red bumps with lines radiating out, resembling a spider's legs) may be symptoms of a liver disease. If a skin problem is suspected of being symptomatic of something else, the first step in an investigation is for the physician to take a blood sample. Blood tests done in general practice would include tests for anemia and kidney, liver, and thyroid function and tests to look for autoimmune diseases. Samples of blood are sent to the laboratory at the local hospital for analysis. The test results are returned to the doctor, who may be able to treat the identified problem directly or alternatively will refer the patient to a specialist.

A fungus responsible for ringworm
A seven-week growth of one of the fungi responsible for ringworm on the scalp (tinea capita). The fungus, Trichophyton violaceum, causes round scaly lesions that itch and cause patches of hair loss.

Investigation of infection

If the doctor suspects that a skin condition is caused by infection, he or she may send tiny samples of skin to a hospital laboratory to find out whether there are bacteria, viruses, or fungi present. Samples are generally collected by rubbing a sterile swab, like a cotton swab, across the affected area. In the case of fungal infections such as ringworm (tinea), the doctor may take scrapings from affected skin, nail clippings, or a few hairs from the scalp.

Glass slide test

This is also called a diascopy. A glass slide or clear plastic spoon pressed onto the affected area of the skin causes the small blood vessels in the skin to constrict so that the amount of blood within the skin is temporarily reduced, revealing whether redness in the skin is caused by vessel dilation or bleeding into the skin and revealing the true color of a lesion. Hopefully, this will aid in a correct diagnosis of the condition. Vasculitis (inflammation of blood vessels, see page 154), tuberculosis, and meningococcal septicemia are examples of conditions that prompt this type of test.

TESTS AT THE HOSPITAL

When a family doctor is unable to make a diagnosis, the patient is referred to the dermatology department of the local hospital. Facilities there enable a wider variety of tests to be carried out.

SKIN BIOPSY

There are two main types of skin biopsies: punch biopsy and scalpel biopsy. Before either test, the area around the site of the biopsy is anesthetized using a local anesthetic injection such as lidocaine.

- A punch biopsy involves removing a cylinder of skin a tenth of an inch wide with a sharp instrument that bores a small hole into the skin. The sample is lifted and put into a preservative, then sent to a histopathologist for

More than 2.5 million skin biopsies are carried out every year in the U.S.

Wood's light test

Wood's light is ultraviolet (UV) filtered through a nickel oxide prism. When Wood's light is shone on skin infected by certain fungi or bacteria, the skin becomes fluorescent.

a and **b** Scalp ringworm arising from fungi belonging to the *Microsporum* genus gives rise to blue-green fluorescence. Some other fungal skin conditions produce yellow fluorescence.

c and **d** The chronic bacterial infection erythrasma fluoresces coral pink—as shown here in a typical site between two toes.

In addition, areas of the skin where pigmentation is absent (see vitiligo, pages 154–155) show up more clearly when bathed in Wood's light.

analysis. The cut on the skin is stitched or sealed with a diathermy needle.

- A scalpel biopsy is performed when a sample of tissue is required that is large enough to enable a comparison of normal and abnormal tissue. An ellipse of skin (shaped like an oval) that includes the area in question is removed, and the skin edges are then stitched together.
- A shave biopsy is very common and is performed by taking a very superficial slice of skin with a scalpel or razor blade. No stitches are required.

PHOTOGRAPHY

If there is concern that a mole is growing or changing, a digital photo may be taken and filed with the patient's medical notes as a record to be compared with the appearance of the mole at the patient's next checkup.

IMMUNOLOGICAL TESTS

Immunological tests examine the body's immune system, which helps protect the body from harmful microorganisms in order to investigate infections, allergies, and irritants. They are very useful in the identification of skin ailments and provide information that is often very valuable when it comes to deciding on the most appropriate treatment.

Skin prick tests

These identify which substance is triggering an immediate allergic response in a patient. They are also used to investigate the itchy red rash urticaria (see page 154). The results are not always helpful, though, because some patients show false positive or false negative results.

A patient must not take antihistamine medication for 48 hours before the test because this will alter the test results. Single drops of commercially prepared dilute antigens are placed on the skin and the skin beneath each drop is pricked with a needle. The drops are then removed with a tissue, and ten minutes later the skin is examined for weals; any red, itchy patches or weals indicate a positive result. Skin prick tests are not performed if there is a risk of the patient experiencing a severe anaphylactic reaction.

Patch tests

These are used to establish whether a patient has contact dermatitis—that is, whether a rash is an allergic response brought on by contact with one or more substances. Drops from a standard selection of "common culprit" allergens are placed on small aluminium disks set within a wide strip of adhesive tape. Disks and tape are then stuck

A patch test for contact dermatitis
This young woman has four allergy test strips on her back. On each test strip are ten disks, or "patches," each of which tests for skin sensitivity to a different allergen. If the skin underneath a patch becomes inflamed, this indicates that the patient is allergic to the substance under the patch.

to the patient's back, so that the allergens come in contact with the skin. If a particular chemical that is not on the standard list is suspected, it will also be included.

The patches are left in place for 48 hours and then are removed after each site has been carefully marked. Inspection at this time will show positive tests as red, swollen, and even covered in blisters. The skin is inspected again after 96 hours, to see whether any further tests have come up positive (these are late responses). If any were positive at 48 hours but are negative at 96 hours, they are considered irritant reactions.

If it is suspected that a rash has been provoked by exposure to ultraviolet (UV) light, more specialized photopatch testing may be available to check this out. Two sets of the same allergens are applied to the skin as above. Then, after the disks have been removed, one set of allergens is exposed to a controlled dose of UV radiation.

Radioallergosorbent test (RAST)

A sample of the patient's blood is taken and sent to a laboratory, where it is tested for evidence of allergies to certain foods or environmental allergens such as the dust mite. A RAST test is performed on its own or with a skin prick test to see whether they both produce the same results.

Immunofluorescence

This is a test used to differentiate among various types of blistering diseases of the skin, such as bullous pemphigoid, pemphigus (see pages 149–150), and dermatitis herpetiformis (see page 138). These disorders are caused by the body reacting against its own tissues. Freshly cut skin sections are treated with an antibody and labeled with fluorescein, a dye that can be seen in UV light. The sample is then examined using UV light, and the location of the antibody on the cell membrane gives diagnostic information about which particular skin disease is present.

LYMPHOSCINTIGRAPHY

This is primarily used to investigate the cause of swelling in the lower legs to determine whether the cause is blockages within the lymphatic channels or the veins, but it can also be used to assess the spread of cancers such as lymphomas affecting the skin (see mycosis fungoides, page 148) and malignant melanoma (see page 147). A radioactive dye is injected into a small lymphatic vessel close to the surface of the foot, and then a scanner is used to track the progress of the dye up the leg and into the lymph nodes in the groin, and beyond if necessary.

Mycosis fungoides
This transmission electron micrograph image shows a slice through cancerous white blood cells (lymphocytes) from a patient with mycosis fungoides. This condition primarily affects the lymphatic system, but it manifests itself as red scaly patches on the skin that resemble those caused by eczema and psoriasis.

CURRENT TREATMENTS

The many treatments for diseases and disorders of the skin can be broadly divided into two categories: those designed to treat large areas and those that enable pinpoint accuracy in order to remove tiny growths and other lesions without damaging the skin around them. Creams and lotions can cover extensive areas, as can phototherapy. When skin has been badly damaged, skin grafting is sometimes required. Doctors freeze, scrape, shave, or burn off many types of benign growths and markings—or even vaporize them with a laser. For life-threatening malignant melanomas, however, the preferred option is still to cut out the tumor and surrounding tissue with a scalpel.

Light treatments

Specialists use laser light and ultraviolet light therapies—alone or in combination with drugs—to treat a variety of skin ailments, from chronic conditions such as psoriasis to cancers of the skin.

TOPICAL PHOTODYNAMIC THERAPY (PDT)

Topical photodynamic therapy is used to treat a variety of premalignant skin lesions and is currently being tested in the treatment of some malignant tumors. First, a cream that contains a light-sensitive drug is spread onto the area of skin to be treated. A few hours later, a light (generally laser light) is shone onto this area; the light is set at a particular wavelength that will react with the photosensitizing drug in the cream. Together, the light and the drug work to destroy the unwanted cells.

This technique is useful for treating areas of skin that have a number of lesions that need to be removed, as can be the case with premalignant skin conditions such as actinic (solar) keratoses (see page 134) and Bowen's disease (pages 136–137).

A new development in topical PDT
The Paterson lamp is a new and potentially more convenient alternative to laser light when carrying out topical photodynamic therapy. The lamp uses lenses and fiberoptics to produce an intense light from an electric current.

Photodynamic therapy is not yet as widely available as it might be, and it does not have the backup data on long-term effectiveness enjoyed by other treatments. But PDT is a particularly useful way of treating areas of skin that might heal poorly after other treatments, such as skin on the lower legs. Other advantages are minimal scarring and reduced risk of infection compared with other treatments.

ULTRAVIOLET PHOTOTHERAPY

Many patients with inflammatory skin disorders observe that their skin improves significantly if they spend time outside exposed to the ultraviolet (UV) radiation in natural sunlight. With the therapeutic benefits of UV in mind, treatments have been devised that provide patients with an artificial source of UV radiation, thereby improving their skin conditions. These treatments are carried out in outpatient offices.

PUVA therapy for psoriasis

a One of the conditions for which ultraviolet phototherapy is particularly effective is psoriasis. This skin condition is characterized by a rapid turnover of skin cells, resulting in red patches covered with silvery scales. Ultraviolet phototherapy comes into play when the psoriasis has become resistant to drugs applied topically as creams or when there is a large area of skin requiring treatment.

b After six weeks of PUVA sessions, the skin has cleared up dramatically. However, PUVA treatment cannot be continued at this level indefinitely because of the risk of premature skin aging and of skin cancer. Therefore, because the underlying causes of the disorder remain, it is likely that the psoriasis will return at a future date.

UVB phototherapy

Regular exposure to artificial UVB light rays administered by a lamp can be a very effective way of managing a number of diseases of the skin, particularly psoriasis. Careful monitoring is vital because UVB tans the skin and too much can burn it; also, as with sunlight, excessive exposure can cause the skin to age prematurely and increase the chances of developing skin cancer. A factor in deciding whether or not to choose UVB phototherapy is whether the patient is fair-skinned and therefore burns easily. Typically, UVB therapy is first given three times a week for six weeks, and then the patient's condition is reviewed and a "maintenance program" is devised.

PUVA therapy

A more potent form of light treatment is PUVA. This combines taking the drug, psoralen and UVA phototherapy. (P plus UVA forms the acronym PUVA.) The drug is usually taken by mouth, although it is sometimes applied in the form of a lotion to allow small areas of the body to

be treated specifically. Two hours later, the skin is exposed to UVA radiation from a fluorescent lamp. The UVA light enhances the effect of the drug on cells in the skin.

There is no doubt that PUVA therapy is a very effective treatment for psoriasis in particular and also for eczema and other less common skin conditions. It can be used to treat mycosis fungoides, a low-grade cancer of the immune system that affects the skin (see page 148). Treatment is generally required twice weekly for about six weeks.

As with any treatment involving exposure to UV radiation, PUVA can produce a sunburn-like reaction. Patients taking psoralen in tablet form find that their skin becomes very sensitive to light in the hours after a treatment session, so they have to cover up from the sun and wear sunglasses. There is also a risk of skin cancer, particularly for patients who need repeat treatments of PUVA over a long period of time. (Because the risk of carcinoma of the penis, male genitalia should be covered during treatment.) As a result of this cancer risk, PUVA treatment is carefully monitored and tends to be prescribed only after UVB phototherapy has been ineffective for some reason.

Drugs for skin problems

There are a number of topical and systemic treatments for acne, eczema, and psoriasis—the prevalent skin problems in society today— as well as treatments to cure or soothe a range of bacterial, viral, and fungal infections, sunburn, and the effects of chemotherapy on the skin.

Drugs can be administered topically (locally) directly to the part of the body requiring treatment or systemically— that is in such a way that the body as a whole is affected (as with tablets and medicines taken by mouth). Topical drugs designed to treat the skin consist of a "vehicle," also called a base, in which there is usually some kind of active ingredient. Vehicles include the following: lotions, thicker "shake lotions" such as calamine, creams, gels, ointments, and pastes. Vehicles hydrate the skin, and they can have an antiinflammatory effect and help the active drug penetrate the skin.

The advantage of topical drug treatment is that the drug is delivered directly to the skin with minimal risk of side effects affecting the body as a whole. However, to be truly effective, the drug must be able to penetrate the skin's outermost layers. Its ability to do this is influenced by a variety of factors:
• the drug itself and its concentration
• the age and existing degree of hydration of the skin
• the type of vehicle

A soothing cream for itchy skin
Emollients are an important part of the treatment of many skin conditions. Regular applications of an emollient to the problem area— in this case an itchy blistering rash caused by contact dermatitis—help keep the skin soothed, smoothed, flexible, and hydrated.

If a topical preparation is used correctly for an appropriate period of time but does not produce the desired effect, a doctor may consider prescribing systemic therapy.

PSORIASIS
Psoriasis (see page 151) is characterized by patches of flaking skin. Treatment aims to relieve inflammation and scaling and to reduce the area of skin involved. The choice of treatment depends on which part of the body is affected, how much skin is affected, and how well the condition and its various treatments are tolerated. Topical therapy is the mainstay for mild to moderate psoriasis, but systemic or other specialist treatments are prescribed in severe cases.

Topical therapies for psoriasis
• **Calcipotriol and tacalcitol** are synthetic vitamin D preparations that block abnormal division of skin cells, increase cell maturation, and modify the immune response that causes inflammation. For many doctors, they are the first choice of topical treatment for psoriasis.

Dovobet: a breakthrough in the treatment of psoriasis

Dovobet is a new topical drug treatment for psoriasis sufferers in the U.K. that is the most significant advance in the treatment of this condition in the last decade. It combines two active ingredients already being used separately to treat psoriasis: calcipotriol and betamethasone. Calcipotriol is a derivative of vitamin D that slows down the excessive production of skin cells that characterizes psoriasis. Betamethasone is a corticosteroid that reduces inflammation. Dovobet comes in ointment form and is applied twice daily for up to four weeks. Improvement in the patient's condition is generally fast and dramatic, often removing the need for phototherapy or systemic drug therapy.

- An emollient may be all that is needed in mild cases.
- Coal tar preparations are available as creams, pastes, and bath additives and may be used up to three times a day. However, they can smell unpleasant and be messy to use. Tar products can also stain skin temporarily and clothes and bedding permanently.
- Salicylic acid is often mixed with other ingredients such as coal tar and dithranol to make a topical preparation. It loosens and removes thick scaly patches.
- Tazarotene is a derivative of vitamin A. It can be used to treat mild to moderate psoriasis where up to a tenth of the body surface area is affected. It irritates the skin a lot, which limits its usefulness. Women who may become pregnant must use adequate contraception during treatment because tazarotene can cause deformities in fetuses.
- Dithranol is an effective topical preparation for psoriasis but must be used carefully because it can severely irritate the skin and permanently stains clothing and bedding. The drug is initially used at a low strength with the concentration slowly increased during a course of treatment. It is applied as a cream, ointment, or paste to affected skin only and then is removed after an hour or less. Dithranol slows down the rapid rate of cell division that causes skin thickening. It is often combined with coal tar or salicylic acid.
- Topical corticosteroids (often just called steroids) may be used in difficult cases for short periods only. They can help with skinfold areas and to counter irritation caused by dithranol.

Systemic drugs for psoriasis

A small number of people do not respond to topical treatment or relapse very quickly afterward. Systemic treatment under specialist supervision may include the use of the vitamin A derivative acitretin, the anticancer drug methotrexate, or the immunosuppressant cyclosporine.

ECZEMA

Most people with atopic (hereditary) dermatitis or eczema are treated with topical therapies.

Topical therapies for eczema

Topical therapies for eczema have three aims: healing the skin, preventing flare-ups, and treating any symptoms.

Psoriasis affects 7 million people in the United States and 1.5 million in the UK.

- Emollients and moisturizers smooth the surface of dry skin and help the skin retain its moisture and become soft, smooth, and flexible. When used correctly, they can allow use of a lower dose of corticosteroid without reducing its effect. Available as lotions, creams, ointments, soap substitutes, and bath oils, they need to be used frequently to be effective.
- Topical corticosterids are used to control flare-ups of eczema. They inhibit the production and action of chemicals that cause inflammation in the skin, thereby reducing inflammation and itching. The steroid must be of a suitable potency for the area to be treated, and it must be applied sparingly, with use limited to the shortest time needed for a clinically acceptable effect. Skin thinning and stretch marks can appear with chronic use, and hypersensitivity to ingredients may lead to symptoms becoming worse.

Systemic drugs for eczema

- Oral corticosteroids are occasionally prescribed to quickly control a severe flare-up of eczema. They are usually taken in high initial doses, which are then reduced every few days over a course of 3 to 4 weeks. As the dose is reduced, topical steroids are increasingly used to counteract the disease flare-up that can occur on withdrawal of the oral steroids.
- Antibiotics may be used when eczema is infected. The most commonly implicated organism is Staphylococcus aureus (staph), which can be treated with oral antibiotics for 7 to 10 days. Flucloxacillin is effective in 90 percent of staph infections. Erythromycin is useful for people who are allergic to penicillin. Recurrent infections can be treated with antiseptic bath oils and emollients. Topical antibiotics should be used only under supervision; short courses cause no problems, but prolonged use can lead to drug resistance.
- Antihistamines of the older, sedating type may help at night if itching is preventing sleep. Because the itch of eczema is not caused by histamine release, nonsedating antihistamines should not be used.
- Evening Primrose oil (gamma linoleic acid) is a controversial treatment with conflicting evidence about

How corticosteroids affect inflamed skin

a Skin becomes inflamed when irritation of skin by allergens and other irritants provokes the release of inflammatory mediators (chemicals that cause inflammation) from white blood cells. These chemicals cause blood vessels close to the skin's surface to dilate, making skin hot, swollen, and red.

b Corticosteroids (also called steroids) are applied to the inflamed skin and absorbed, resulting in inhibition of the inflammatory mediators. Blood vessels return to normal and as a result the swelling, redness, and heat of the skin is reduced.

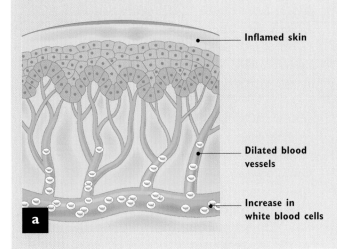

Inflamed skin

Dilated blood vessels

Increase in white blood cells

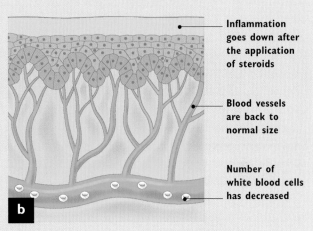

Inflammation goes down after the application of steroids

Blood vessels are back to normal size

Number of white blood cells has decreased

its efficacy. For patients with very dry skin it can be a very effective way of reducing dryness and inflammation in the skin.

TREATING ACNE

Response to treatment is relatively slow, and patients need to realize that it may take up to six months before they see a significant improvement in their condition. But it is very important that a patient carefully maintains the prescribed treatment regimen: Poor compliance can lead to bacterial resistance and significantly reduce the effectiveness of the treatment.

Topical therapies for acne

Topical therapies remain the mainstay for the treatment of mild acne. They include drugs that influence the growth and function of acne bacteria and inflammation—known as comedone formation.

- **Benzoyl peroxide** has antibacterial properties. Benzoyl peroxide treats inflamed and noninflamed skin effectively, but it can cause irritation and bleaching.
- **Topical antibiotics** are helpful in reducing inflammatory acne lesions like papules (small raised bumps) and

pustules. Clindamycin and erythromycin are common choices.
- **Topical retinoids** (adapalene, isotretinoin, tretinoin) are anti-comedonal therapies that are most effective in reducing blackheads and whiteheads. A common side effect is skin irritation. Alternating use of topical antibiotics and topical retinoids can produce good results. Patients using topical retinoids should avoid excessive UV light.
- **Topical combination preparations** include antibiotics and antiinflammatory agents such as erythromycin plus benzoyl peroxide or zinc. These combination preparations appear to induce less bacterial resistance than the use of topical antibiotics alone.

Systemic drugs for acne

Oral therapies for acne can be divided into three groups: antibiotics, hormonal therapies, and retinoids (the best known of which is isotretinoin).
- **Antibiotics** taken orally have been the mainstay of treatment for inflammatory acne for years. They are antiinflammatory and reduce the activity of acne bacteria. Studies have shown that minocycline is

the most effective drug, followed by doxycycline, trimethoprim, oxytetracycline, and erythromycin. A major concern with the use of systemic antibiotics is the development of resistance of acne bacteria to the antibiotics. Combining topical benzoyl peroxide with oral antibiotics can reduce the risk of this.

- **Hormonal therapy** with the anti-androgen drug spironolactone is used because androgen hormones control sebum production. Spironolactone is also a diuretic used to treat heart failure, liver disease, and high blood pressure.
- **Isotretinoin** is effective in treating all mechanisms responsible for acne. It is only available from dermatologists and is used for severe and otherwise nonresponsive acne. The most important side effect is the possibility of abnormal development of a fetus, so fertile women must use adequate contraception while taking the drug and for four weeks after treatment. Other side effects include very dry lips and dry facial skin, which can be minimized by regular use of lip balm and oil-free moisturizers. Isotretinoin may also have psychological effects on patients, causing depression and mood changes. Patients—and their parents—must be advised of these risks prior to treatment.

The herpes simplex virus
This colored transmission electron micrograph image shows the herpes simplex virus, which is responsible for cold sores and genital herpes. The virus causes small fluid-filled blisters on the skin.

TREATING SKIN INFECTIONS
Bacteria, viruses, and fungi may all be responsible for triggering skin infections.

Bacterial skin infections
- **Impetigo** is a skin infection caused by Stapylococcus or Streptococcus. It leads to the formation of small pustules. Early treatment with antibiotics such as penicillin or a cephalosporin can prevent a deeper skin infection from developing.
- **Folliculitis, boils, and carbuncles** can be prevented from spreading by keeping the skin clean with an antibacterial soap. Antibiotics are used for boils and carbuncles.
- **Erysipelas** is treated with the antibiotics penicillin or erythromycin.
- **Cellulitis** needs prompt treatment to keep the infection from spreading rapidly and reaching the blood. It is often treated with penicillin or a penicillin-type drug. Patients with mild cellulitis may take oral antibiotics, but older people and those with a serious infection usually receive antibiotics by injection before they take oral antibiotics.

Viral skin infections
- **Herpes simplex** causes the viral infection of the lips known as a cold sore, as well as genital herpes. The affected area should be kept clean by gentle washing with soap and water, then carefully dried. Antiviral creams such as acyclovir and penciclovir are sometimes effective when placed directly on blisters. They do not cure herpes simplex, but they shorten the duration of symptoms by a few days.
- **Herpes zoster** is the virus that causes shingles. No drug can eliminate the virus, but antivirals such as acyclovir or famciclovir can be given by mouth for a short period of skin eruption.

• Human papillomavirus causes warts. Treatment depends on the location, type, and severity of the wart, and how long it has been on the skin. Most common warts disappear without treatment within two years. Daily application of solutions or bandages containing salicylic and lactic acids soften the infected skin, which can be peeled off to make the wart disappear faster. A doctor can freeze the wart with liquid nitrogen (see page 119) or can use electrodesiccation (page 120) or laser surgery (page 126). A wart can also be treated with the chemicals trichloroacetic acid or cantharidin; the wart is destroyed, but sometimes new warts crop up around the edges of the old one.

Fungal skin infections

• **Topical agents** are in most cases the first-line treatment for superficial

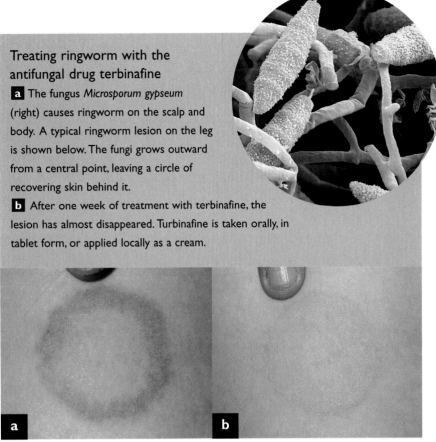

Treating ringworm with the antifungal drug terbinafine

a The fungus *Microsporum gypseum* (right) causes ringworm on the scalp and body. A typical ringworm lesion on the leg is shown below. The fungi grows outward from a central point, leaving a circle of recovering skin behind it.

b After one week of treatment with terbinafine, the lesion has almost disappeared. Turbinafine is taken orally, in tablet form, or applied locally as a cream.

fungal infections. Topical therapies avoid the potentially serious side effects of systemic treatments. Creams include miconazole (sold as Micatin) and ketoconazole (Nizoral), both of which cause the loss of fungal cell membrane integrity and activity and stop fungal growth. Topical terbinafine kills the fungus. The principal side effects of such topical agents are local irritation and sensitivity reactions. Treatment generally lasts 4 to 6 weeks and may need to be continued beyond the clearing of symptoms.

• **Systemic therapy** may be required for chronic infections and for disabling or extensive disease in patients with compromised immune systems or who are intolerant or unresponsive to topical treatment. Oral therapy is the preferred treatment for fungal nail infections and for fungal infections of the scalp and beard area. The site of infection and the identity of the fungus determines the choice of oral agent. The drug terbinafine is frequently prescribed; it accumulates well in skin tissue and kills fungi, is well-tolerated, and interacts with few other drugs. If the yeastlike fungus Candida is involved in the infection, then a drug such as fluconazole (sold as Diflucan) is an appropriate oral agent. In cases that do

not respond to fluconazole, a similar drug called itraconazole (Sporanox) may sometimes be effective. Griseofulvin is the oldest of the oral antifungal agents. It is now only used for ringworm of the scalp in children.

SUNBURN

There are a number of remedies useful for relieving the pain of hot and sunburned skin. Taking a lukewarm bath or shower can help cool the skin. Exposure to sun dries out the skin; smoothing an emollient onto the skin or adding one to the water in a bath helps soften the skin and conserve moisture within the epidermis. It is not essential to use a special "aftersun" lotion—any cooling emollient will work. Calamine lotion, applied often and liberally to the burned area, will cool the skin as it dries, but it must not be used on broken skin.

An oral antihistamine may help with itching. Lotions, sprays, or creams containing antihistamines or local anesthetics should not be used on the skin because they can cause the skin to become sensitized and develop an eczema-like rash. Topical steroids will often reduce inflammation in sunburned skin.

How medication can affect skin and hair

Skin can react adversely to medications for many different kinds of ailments. Itching and rashes are the most common symptoms. In addition, hair loss may be triggered by reactions to drugs taken to fight a variety of diseases and disorders.

WHEN DRUGS CAUSE A SKIN PROBLEM

Skin reactions to medication may be caused by several different mechanisms; in many cases, the exact mechanism is unknown. Hypersensitivity reactions are the most common causes of drug rashes. Other causes are photosensitivity, accumulation of the drug in the skin, or exacerbation of a preexisting skin condition.

Symptoms of skin hypersensitivity reactions include itches and rashes, and also wheezing and anaphylaxis (shocklike symptoms brought on by a sudden histamine release). Drugs responsible include aspirin, antibiotics (especially penicillins, cephalosporins, and sulfonamides), antiepileptics, allopurinol, and gold. Most rashes clear up a week or so after the patient stops taking the drug that is the cause.

Drugs that cause photosensitivity rashes triggered by sunlight include antibacterials such as tetracyclines and sulfonamides; diuretics, such as thiazides; drugs for irregular heart beats, such as amiodarone; and anti-psychotics like phenothiazines. Patients taking these medicines are likely to need a high-SPF product for extra protection before going out into the sun.

WHEN DRUGS CAN CAUSE HAIR LOSS

Chemotherapy drugs damage normal cells as well as cancer cells. Healthy cells that are affected often include those in hair follicles, sometimes resulting in temporary hair loss. If hair loss occurs, it usually begins within a few weeks of starting treatment. The amount of hair lost depends on the combination of drugs taken, the dose, and the way the individual's body reacts to the drugs. Loss of hair from the scalp may be partial or complete and eyebrows, eyelashes, and body and pubic hair may also be lost.

With some chemotherapy drugs, wearing a specially designed "cold cap" before, during, and after each treatment session prevents hair loss by temporarily reducing the flow of blood to the scalp and thereby the amount of anticancer drug that reaches the hair follicles and by slowing the metabolism of the follicles, making them less susceptible to damage. A number of other drugs can cause hair loss, including antithyroid drugs, anticoagulants, and certain combination contraceptive pills.

Tips for hair while undergoing chemotherapy

- If the chemotherapy is likely to cause hair loss, get your hair cut short before treatment begins and use gentle hair products.
- Try not to comb or brush your hair too roughly—use a soft brush.
- Do not perm your hair during chemotherapy or for 12 weeks after treatment.
- Use only mild vegetable-based colorants—check with a hairdresser or chemotherapy nurse.
- Do not use heated styling products, including hairdryers.

If severe hair loss does occur, a patient who feels self-conscious about it can try wearing a scarf or hat when going out, or ask the chemo nurse or doctor about a wig.

Basic surgical treatments

There are a lot of ways to remove unwanted or potentially harmful growths from the surface of the skin. Treatments range from cutting to freezing to burning, with bleeding stopped at the source by cauterization.

Cryotherapy to remove a wart
A wart on a finger is being treated with liquid nitrogen on a cotton swab. The liquid nitrogen freezes the wart solid. As the wart thaws, a blister forms and the wart is shed with the resulting scab.

CRYOTHERAPY

The use of cold to kill tissue is known as cryotherapy or cryosurgery. This is a widely used treatment for a range of dermatological problems. It involves the application of a freezing agent to the affected skin. The agent causes damaged cells to burst and die because of the rapid freezing and then thawing that takes place.

The most common freezing agent used today is liquid nitrogen. The liquid nitrogen is applied for 10 to 20 seconds to the site of the lesion, using either a spray gun from a distance of about a half-inch or a cotton swab.

Typical conditions that can be treated in this way include warts, freckles, liver spots on the back of hands, and some skin precancers and cancers.

Cryotherapy can be quite painful and will cause inflammation and in some cases blistering. Sometimes a mild painkiller is needed to relieve discomfort caused by swollen and inflamed skin. Occasionally, cryotherapy can cause mild scarring or a permanent change in color of the treated skin, especially in dark-skinned patients.

CURETTAGE

Another technique that allows the removal of simple skin lesions is curettage. A local anesthetic is injected into the skin, and then the skin lesion is scraped off with a sharp-edged curette spoon. The base of the skin, now raw and oozing or bleeding, is sealed by cauterisation.

Curettage is only possible if the material being scraped off is more frail than the surrounding skin or when there is a natural cleavage plane between the lesion and the normal tissue that surrounds it. The resulting shallow wound heals by a combination of wound shrinkage and skin rejuvenation.

Using this method, a number of lesions can be treated in a relatively short period of time. The final cosmetic results can be excellent, and there is very little postoperative discomfort. The disadvantage of curettage as a technique is that because the lesion is simply being

EXPERIENCING CURETTAGE

A small nodule that bled easily and frequently developed on the side of one of my toes. My doctor referred me to a dermatologist to have it looked at.

The dermatologist told me that it was nothing to worry about: It was a pyogenic granuloma, which can appear after skin has been cut or damaged in some way. He sent me to another doctor to have it removed.

First, the doctor cleaned the area around the granuloma. Then she injected a local anesthetic between two toes. After the anesthetic had taken effect, she scooped out the growth with a tiny curette spoon and applied an electrically heated wire to the cut skin to seal the tiny wound and prevent any bleeding. And that was it. The procedure was painless throughout and took about 10 minutes, most of which was spent waiting for the local anesthetic to work.

scraped off the top layer of skin, there is always a small but recognizable risk that the lesion may recur.

ELECTROCAUTERY

Electrocautery is a very neat way of stopping any bleeding on the skin's surface. A wire is heated by electrical conduction to sufficiently produce enough heat to burn and thereby destroy the cut blood vessels and put an end to bleeding from an incision in the skin. This technique is also used to burn away warts and other growths on the surface of the skin.

ELECTROSURGERY

Electrosurgery involves the use of an electric current to cut or burn tissue in a controlled manner. It is most frequently used to cut away lesions of various kinds. There are different methods suitable for different conditions and situations.

- **Cutting diathermy** is a technique that uses an electric knife—a diathermy knife, actually an electrode—to cut tissues. There is very little bleeding from capillaries because the cut edges are immediately cauterized. Sometimes a diathermy snare or needle is used instead.
- **Electrofulguration** destroys tissue with sparks sprayed from an electrode that is not actually touching the lesion, thus keeping destruction and scarring to a minimum. It is used to remove small skin growths such as nodules and warts.

Electrocautery on the back of a hand
Electrocautery is taking place here in order to clean, seal, and neaten a wound after a shave excision. A shave excision is used for the removal of benign growths such as skin tags. The growth is shaved off the skin with minimal disturbance to the skin below it.

- **Electrodesiccation** involves touching a lesion with an electrode, causing slightly deeper tissue destruction. It is often followed by curettage. This method can remove a wide variety of small growths. One use is the treatment of eyelid xanthelasma (see page 155) by removing the little fatty deposits that can develop around the eyes.
- **Electrolysis** is employed to remove unwanted terminal hairs. A needle is passed into the hair follicle, and an electric current is used to destroy the hair root.

SKIN EXCISION

When removing a mole or other growth from the surface of the skin by means of surgical excision, the same procedure is followed as for a scalpel biopsy (see page 108). The surgeon begins by drawing an ellipse on the skin's surface around the area to be removed. The ellipse is generally about three times as long as it is wide. The skin is cleaned, and local anesthetic is administered. The surgeon uses a scalpel to cut along the two curved lines that make up the ellipse, as far down as the layer of subcutaneous fat. The growth and the skin surrounding it are removed and the two cut surfaces are stitched together; generally only a few stitches are needed.

SURGICAL REMOVAL OF SKIN TAGS

Snip excision is a simple technique for the removal of small skin tags. The stalk of the skin tag is held away from the skin and snipped off at its base by a pair of sharp scissors. This often results in a spontaneous end in bleeding. There is usually no need for a local anesthetic unless a larger skin tag requires bleeding to be stopped with a stitch or cauterization.

REMOVING A LIPOMA

A lipoma is a benign tumor made up of fat cells; it shows up as a lump below the skin. If it is unsightly or causing discomfort, it can be removed by means of a simple excision of the fat through a cut in the overlying skin. The only disadvantage of this procedure is that there is the potential to produce a rather large scar. To keep the incision (and resulting scar) to a minimum, the lipoma may be broken up into smaller pieces before being brought out through the incision made in the skin. Alternatively, the fat within the lipoma can be fragmented and removed by the procedure known as liposuction (see page 99).

Skin grafts and transplants

Skin grafting involves taking healthy skin from one part of the body and placing it over a damaged area of skin instead. A graft allows injured skin to heal more quickly and effectively and with less scarring than would otherwise be the case.

WHEN IS A SKIN GRAFT NEEDED?

A skin graft is required when a defect in the skin is so large that it is not amenable to natural healing or closure with stitches. Such a defect has usually been caused by a burn or other injury or by surgery (to remove a skin lesion, for example). One treatment option is having a flap of skin brought over from a neighboring area and grafted onto the defect. Alternatively, skin from a site elsewhere is transplanted to the damaged area—this is a straightforward skin graft.

MAKING A FLAP

A flap is a patch of skin that has been mostly cut away from the body but left attached at one end so that its blood and nerve supply is retained. The free end of the flap is stitched into the area to be repaired, and when the flap has healed in place (a process that takes 2 to 3 weeks), the flap is cut free from its source and fully sewn in.

- A local flap uses skin that lies right next to the area to be covered. Sometimes the adjacent skin is stretched before it is used as a flap; this is done by inserting a balloonlike device under the skin beside the area to be covered and then slowly allowing the balloon to expand. This process is called tissue expansion. Because the skin of a local flap already has an intact blood supply and is similar to the skin that has been removed, the final result is often far superior to a more traditional skin graft, and there is a much smaller chance of the new skin failing to "take."
- A regional flap uses skin that is not right beside the area that requires a skin graft. The flap is stitched in place but remains attached to its original source by a narrow neck of tissue called a pedicle until the flap has healed into its new site. The pedicle is then removed.

SKIN GRAFTS

There are two main types of skin graft: a full thickness skin graft that includes the epidermis and the dermis below it and a split thickness skin graft in which only the epidermis and upper dermis are used as a graft.

A full thickness skin graft

A month after surgery to remove a squamous cell carcinoma (see page 131), skin is taken from another site to replace the skin lost from the patient's nose.

a The donor site for the skin graft is just below the hairline, in front of an ear. Scarring in this area will not be noticeable.

b The donor skin is grafted over the scarred nostril. In this picture, the skin graft has been in place for one week and the stitches are about to be taken out.

c Four weeks after surgery, the new graft has healed very well. The pink coloring should fade with time.

Full thickness skin graft

A full thickness skin graft is the best choice when cosmetic appearance (on the face, for example) or the ability to withstand wear and tear (as with the palm of the hand) are important factors. There is a limit to how much skin can be taken from the donor site, however, because skin at the donor site will not grow back: Instead, the cut edges are stitched together to close the wound.

The surgeon tries to match skin from the donor site as closely as possible to the skin at the recipient site; sites chosen are generally free of terminal hairs and have skin to spare (crease of the elbow, for example).

A split thickness skin graft
A skin graft such as the one shown in place here is performed when a wound is too large to be stitched shut or when severe scarring would occur if the wound was left to heal naturally.

Split thickness skin graft

With a split thickness graft, enough of the epidermal appendages (hair follicles and sweat and sebaceous glands) remain at the donor site for the skin to grow back and close the defect made by the graft. Therefore, larger areas of skin can be taken from a donor site than would be possible with a full thickness graft—an entire thigh can be stripped if need be—and so larger areas of damaged skin can be covered than with full thickness skin graft. The skin graft itself is a form of biological dressing: With time, the grafted skin is shed and the patient's own skin regenerates.

The disadvantage is that the donor site can be left very raw and sore for several weeks, until it eventually heals over. (Patients who have undergone split thickness skin grafts often suffer more pain at donor sites than do patients with full thickness skin grafts.) Also, the final result at the recipient site is frequently less satisfactory than after a full thickness graft: The new skin is likely to be less supple, hairless, and worse looking.

Skin is shaved off the donor site using a power dermatome—a surgical instrument that cuts off very thin slices of skin—or a scalpel blade. The donor site most often used is the front of the thighs.

POSSIBLE COMPLICATIONS

- **Graft death** This can occur because of infection, a small bleed below the skin graft, or a poor blood supply to the graft. A poor blood supply may be precipitated by a patient smoking; patients are therefore encouraged to give up smoking a week prior to surgery and for at least two weeks afterward while the graft is taking.
- **Graft may contract** Other complications related to skin grafts include the fact that sometimes the wound area contracts and shrinks in size, pulling on neighboring

tissues and giving the skin a puckered appearance.

- **Sore donor site** For some patients, the main problem is not so much the recipient site but the donor site, which can be sore and uncomfortable for some time after the graft has been removed. For this reason local flaps have an obvious advantage.

SKIN TRANSPLANTS

When a patient has a wound that needs to be covered with skin immediately but there is not enough healthy skin for this job, the patient may receive skin from another donor (living or dead) as a temporary biological dressing. This solution has to be short-term because the patient's body will ultimately reject the "foreign" skin, and the use of immunosuppressive drugs to prevent rejection is not a suitable treatment for someone who has a major skin defect and is therefore wide open to infection. Cadaver skin (generally from the thighs and back) can be stored in a skin bank, if this facility is available. There are about 40 skin tissue banks in the United States that are accredited by the American Association of Tissue Banks.

ON THE CUTTING EDGE

Growing new skin for grafting

One solution to the problem of finding a supply of suitable skin for permanent grafting is to grow new skin. To avoid rejection by the patient's body, the new skin needs to be "grown" from a sample taken from the patient's own body. Scientists can now do this at least for the epidermis. They can take a strip of epidermis the size of a postage stamp and stimulate the cells to multiply, producing a sheet of epidermal skin that can be grafted over the patient's wound. At present, the process is a slow and expensive one, so this treatment is not yet as widely available as doctors would like.

Treatments for burns

When dealing with a burn, the first priority is to prevent infection from invading the damaged area. Healing must then be promoted by whatever means is most appropriate. In serious burns, overcoming shock is often an immediate and pressing concern.

The causes of burns are fire, water (scalding), chemicals, electricity, and UV rays. A burn's seriousness depends on how much of the surface area of the skin is affected and how deeply a burn has penetrated the skin.

SHOCK

Swelling and blistering result from leakage of plasma from blood vessels damaged by a burn. In burns affecting 15 percent or more of skin surface in adults (10 percent in children), loss of plasma impairs the circulation, leading to shock and requiring an immediate blood or saline transfusion to restore the blood volume.

Painkilling drugs are also important, because pain contributes to shock. Loss of nerve endings in the deeper layers of the skin can result in a third-degree burn being less painful than a first or second-degree burn.

INFECTION

An ever-present danger with burns of any sort is infection. Antibiotics are often prescribed to lower the risk of infection.

Different depths of burn

First-degree burn
Affects superficial cells of the epidermis

Superficial second-degree burn
Damages epidermis and upper dermis

Deep second-degree burn
Affects the epidermis and deep dermis

Third-degree burn
The epidermis and dermis are destroyed, and tissues below are affected

SKIN HEALING AND REPAIR

Treatment varies according to the depth and extent of the burn.
- **First-degree burns** may require no special treatment apart from initial cooling of the burn by prolonged immersion in cool, clean water.
- **Second-degree burns** may heal fully, as long as traces of sebaceous and sweat glands and hair follicles remain within the dermis and there

is no extra damage from infection. A dressing will keep the area moist and prevent infection. A topical agent is often applied as well.
- **Third-degree burns** are often severe enough to require a skin graft. The hair follicles and sweat glands have been destroyed, so the skin cannot grow back unless it is able to grow inward from the edges of the wound.

Mesh skin graft
a A piece of skin taken from an unburned donor site on the patient is prepared for a skin graft by being passed through a mesh machine. This enlarges it considerably by turning it into a hexagonal lattice.
b The mesh skin graft is laid over the burn injury and held in place with a dressing. This technique can be used when burns are so extensive that there is not enough healthy skin remaining for a traditional skin graft.

Skin resurfacing

Chemical peels and dermabrasion help smooth out and resurface skin that is less than perfect. Benign skin lesions, extensive acne scarring, uneven pigmentation, skin damage from exposure to too much sun— all can be improved by these treatments.

CHEMICAL PEELS

A chemical peel employs a caustic chemical to destroy the epidermis. The peeling solution is painted onto the skin and then removed after a precisely timed interval. Over the next few days, the dead skin peels away; the skin then heals and the overall result is to give the skin a smoother, tighter, less scarred appearance.

The use of caustic agents on the skin essentially destroys the superficial part of the skin. The epidermis is removed, allowing the chemical to penetrate the upper part of the dermis. The caustic agent also helps stimulate collagen production in the skin.

Chemical peels first came into common use in the 1960s with the introduction of the phenol peel. The main types of caustic agents currently used in peels are trichloracetic acid, alphahydroxy acids, and phenol. Often, a succession of peels is needed to achieve the desired result. The peels are used either alone or in conjunction with dermabrasion or laser rejuvenation treatments.

Chemical treatment for xanthelasma

Fatty deposits around the eye known as xanthelasma can be removed by the application of trichloracetic acid, but care must be taken to protect the eyes from this caustic agent.

The chemical strength of the peeling agent and the time it is left on the skin dictates how deeply the peel penetrates. The greater the depth, the more radical the result. However, the deeper the peel, the greater the recovery time that is needed before the skin has fully healed.

Trichloracetic acid (TCA)

Trichloracetic acid at a concentration of 10 percent left on the skin for several minutes will result in tingling and a little discomfort, some facial redness, and the subsequent sloughing of skin cells from the uppermost layer of the skin. This superficial chemical peeling is used as a quick skin rejuvenating treatment—it can even be fitted into a lunch-hour, if necessary, and is therefore sometimes called a "lunch-time peel."

Removing spider veins

a First, a chemical peel is used to remove the epidermis of the skin on the patient's cheek to prepare the skin for the laser therapy to come.
b Laser treatment then focuses light and heat on the damaged veins —it does not harm the surrounding tissues. When treatment is finished, the cheek is redder than before, but there are fewer visible veins. The redness will subside as the skin heals.

TCA at 30–50 percent provides a medium-depth chemical peel. The deeper penetration of the dermis results in greater bruising, swelling, and redness. Treatment at this level of concentration is an effective way of treating a variety of skin lesions and markings including warts, liver spots, acne scars, and xanthelasma—fatty deposits around the eyes (see page 155).

Alphahydroxy acids (AHAs)
As with trichloracetic acid, peels containing alphahydroxy acids produce a superficial peel in lower concentrations and a medium chemical peel in higher concentrations. They are used for many of the same reasons as trichloracetic acid peels.

Phenol
Phenol produces a deep chemical peel that gives the most dramatic results but requires the longest recovery time. One factor to be aware of is that phenol removes pigmentation, so the treated skin will be permanently paler than untreated skin.

DERMABRASION
Also called dermaplaning or skin planing, this technique involves abrasion of the skin to remove superficial lesions or to soften depressed scars—those from acne for example. It is particularly effective on the face, because regeneration of the epidermis proceeds very quickly on facial skin, thereby allowing rapid healing and reducing the risk of scarring. Although dermabrasion is not used as often as it once was because of the increasing number of other treatments, it remains very effective in the right hands.

How is it done?
The technique involves the use of a high-speed rotary drill with abrasion wheels that plane off skin cells to the mid dermis. A spray refrigerant in effect freezes the skin to allow the rotary drill to pass over the lesions without tearing the skin unnecessarily.

Once skin has been removed, there is some bleeding. This is temporary, however, and healing is usually rapid. Crusting and scabs will form over the planed skin; these eventually fall off to reveal the new, pink skin underneath. There is a risk of infection; therefore, doctors often give their patients preventative treatment in the form of antibiotics. Patients with darker skins risk a permanent change in the pigmentation of skin treated in this way.

Microdermabrasion

Based on traditional dermabrasion but less invasive, less traumatic, and faster healing is microdermabrasion. The treatment improves the appearance of enlarged pores, mild acne scars, uneven pigmentation, and a host of skin defects arising from sun damage.

a In this technique, a "wand" containing abrading crystals is passed over the skin. An integral vacuum sucks up skin debris to exfoliate the skin. No anesthetic is necessary. Using gentle movements, the therapist works the wand over the skin vertically and then horizontally. The vacuum pressure is reduced while she works around the delicate eye area.

b Before treatment by microdermabrasion, this patient's skin shows clear evidence of sun damage.

c After treatment, the condition of the skin has been subtly improved. The comparative gentleness of the treatment means that it cannot be a one-tme solution to skin problems: After a course of four to six 20-minute sessions, follow-up treatments are needed every couple of months to keep the skin in good condition.

Laser treatments for skin conditions

Lasers allow the destruction of the target tissue only, with surrounding tissues remaining intact and bleeding kept to a minimum. In recent years, these advantages have been put to use to treat various lesions and vascular conditions and the effects of sun damage and aging.

Depending on the power, wavelength, exposure time, and tissue being targeted, lasers can have several different effects on the body, hence their use in many different clinical specialties. In dermatology, they are most used for their heat-producing effects.

The type of laser and its optimal wavelength dictate its use: Alexandrite and ruby lasers, for example, target melanin so are used to treat pigment problems; carbon dioxide lasers vaporize tissue and are used in skin resurfacing or cutting; bromide and argon lasers target hemoglobin and are used to treat problems in blood vessels or to heat-seal vessels.

LASERS FOR VASCULAR SKIN CONDITIONS

Conditions that are vascular are those related to or supplied with blood vessels. They include facial thread veins and birthmarks such as port wine stains and strawberry nevi. Lasers to treat vascular conditions target

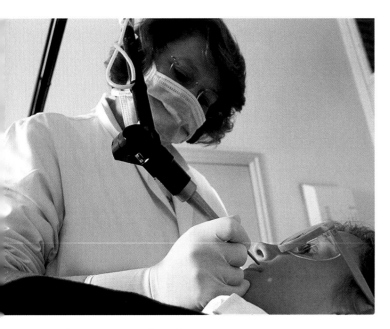

Laser treatment in action
The laser works by focusing extreme light and heat energy on a very small area, vaporizing that area in the process. The energy is emitted from the needle-like device in the middle and is visible as a red dot on the face of the patient.

Is laser therapy the best way of treating spider veins in the legs?

For spider veins—broken blood vessels—in the lower legs, the traditional treatment is sclerotherapy. The veins are injected with sclerosant chemicals that cause the veins to shrivel and close down, thus improving their appearance. In recent years, laser treatments have been introduced, but experience has revealed that laser therapy for spider veins in the legs is not as effective as sclerotherapy.

ASK THE EXPERT

the red of hemoglobin in blood cells, leading to heat generation and the destruction of blood vessels. The first lasers were painful for patients and resulted in bruising. These older lasers have largely been superseded by lasers with associated cooling devices that allow the top layer of the skin to remain undamaged by the heat generated by the laser. Cooling the skin ahead of time and during the procedure also reduces pain for the patient. In addition, these newer lasers produce less bruising and can penetrate deeper into the skin, allowing the treatment of deeper blood vessels or other vascular lesions.

Laser therapy for facial thread veins

Thread veins are broken blood vessels that are visible because they are so close to the skin's surface. The most common cause of facial thread veins is overexposure to ultraviolet (UV) radiation. Facial thread veins used to be treated with electrocautery, but there was always a risk that a patient would be left with a small depressed scar. Today, laser therapy is the preferred treatment. Lasers used to treat vascular skin conditions are very effective in removing facial blood vessels, leaving minimal bruising. However, there is a small risk that the facial thread veins will return in a few years. It may be that this happens when UV rays is the underlying cause, and recurrence occurs with repeated exposure to UV radiation.

Lightening a birthmark

a An increase in the size of blood vessels in the skin results in a port wine stain, an area of permanent flushing. In children, these stains are flat and pink, but they become more purple with age. They may also become more "lumpy," which can make applying camouflage makeup difficult. Treatment using an argon laser can be very successful.

b Up to 10 treatment sessions about 8 weeks apart produce significant skin lightening in up to 90 percent of affected individuals.

ABLATIVE LASERS

Ablative lasers are destructive: They vaporize or remove skin and can also cut tissue quickly and precisely. They can treat blood vessel problems and excess pigmentation, remove warts and skin tags, or resurface the skin following acne, sun damage, or signs of aging. With each pass of the laser over the skin, the skin is removed. Bleeding is kept to a minimum, which limits blood loss and allows the operator a clearer view of the operation site.

The main advantage of laser ablation for skin resurfacing is its success rate: After the top layer of skin is removed and the unblemished skin is left underneath, the appearance of the skin is often dramatically improved. There are many disadvantages, however, including the following:

• Healing can take up to six months.

• The skin can be left with prolonged redness and occasionally some discoloration. Although temporary, this inflammation can be uncomfortable or even painful for patients.

• Patients may be unable to go to work for several weeks after the procedure while the skin is healing.

• Because the skin is raw after surgery, it is prone to infection; often patients are given antibiotics or antiviral treatment to lower the risk of infection.

• Patients with darker skin are often left with permanently discolored skin.

NONABLATIVE LASERS

A nonablative laser, by definition, does not vaporize the skin. These lasers are used at a lower wavelength than ablative models, so they don't produce heat. They can treat facial lines caused by aging and sun damage and also soft scarring. They act by stimulating collagen production, thereby "plumping" the skin up so that slight irregularities are softened and the skin's appearance is improved.

Nonablative lasers have several advantages over conventional resurfacing lasers.

• They may be used on patients of all skin types.

• Because there is no skin ablation, there is no recovery time; sometimes patients have this treatment and go straight back to work.

The disadvantages are that improvements in appearance may take place more slowly and be more subtle.

LASERS FOR OTHER SKIN CONDITIONS

Lasers are also now available to treat pigmented growths such as seborrheic keratoses (basal cell papillomas, see page 135). They have also been modified to remove tattoos as well as pigment changes. Laser tattoo removal has mixed results: Some pigments respond better than others, so a tattoo that is primarily black or blue is fairly easy to remove completely, whereas reds and yellows are more difficult. Laser tattoo removal should not leave any scar.

Mohs micrographic surgery

In the 1950s, Dr. Frederick Mohs developed a technique for excising basal cell carcinomas and similar tumors. Mohs micrographic surgery (MMS) has been refined and improved ever since and is now a sophisticated, widely used technique.

Basal cell carcinoma (BCC) is the most common form of cancer in both the United States and Australia, and it is showing an increase in incidence in the UK. It occurs almost exclusively in white-skinned people, and the most significant causative factor is continued exposure over time to sunlight. For this reason, it occurs mainly in the areas of the body that are exposed—the head, neck, and face. BCCs tend to be relatively slow growing and not to spread to other parts of the body. The aim of treatment is to preserve as much healthy surrounding skin and tissue as possible. It involves the alternate removal and microscopic examination of any tissue harboring cancer cells. It results in the total eradication of the cancer.

This type of surgery is generally performed by specially trained dermatologists. There is an organization of doctors who have advanced training in the Mohs procedures. It is called the American College of Mohs Micrographic Surgery and Cutaneous Oncology, or ACMMSCO or Mohs College for short. Dr. Mohs himself was the first president of the college.

For many plastic surgeons and dermatologists, MMS is the gold standard of treatment for BCCs, particularly those around the eyes and nose. Other treatments—such as cryosurgery, curettage and cautery, radiation, and topical therapy with drugs—may also be used, but they have the disadvantage of not detecting that all cancer cells have been removed. There is, therefore, a significant risk of recurrence. Other cancers that might be treated by MMS include squamous cell carcinomas and some small malignant melanomas.

The procedure—step by step

1 MMS is a good treatment option for a cancer in an area where it is important to preserve healthy tissue for functional and aesthetic reasons, such as around the eyes. The procedure involves alternate surgery and microscopic examination of removed tissue to detect the "roots" of the visible cancer. The patient is given a local anesthetic and may also be sedated.

2 The visible tumor is removed and examined under a microscope. The surgeon builds up a "site map" of the tumor, detecting areas where there are still cancer roots in the skin. Using the "map," the surgeon returns to an area where cancerous cells remain and removes a thin layer of tissue. This is examined under the microscope. If any area of removed tissue still shows signs of cancer, the surgeon returns to that area and removes another thin slice of tissue for microscopic examination. This continues until no cancerous cells can be detected.

3 Removal of only cancerous tissue preserves as much normal tissue as possible, while assuring the surgeon that the horizontal and vertical margins of the incisions are clear of cancer. The surgeon then chooses the best healing option for the patient.

4 The wound heals and is barely noticeable.

Facts about MMS

- The doctor can be sure that all of the cancer cells have been taken away because the whole cancer is excised and examined in its entirety rather than in small sections. This minimizes the chances of false negative results.
- The size of the remaining hole—and hence the scar—will be smaller because the doctor does not have to estimate the extent of the malignant growth.
- The surgery can generally be performed under a local anesthetic in an outpatient clinic, which means that even elderly and frail patients who might not be well enough for a general anesthetic, can benefit from the surgery.
- The surgery is successful, with an overall five-year cure rate of 99 percent.
- Mohs is not suitable for everyone. The most likely candidates have a recurrence of a BCC more than three fourths of an inch in diameter on the eyes, ears, lips, or nose, or on the nose to mouth lines (nasolabial folds). A BCC invading surrounding nerves may also be treated with MMS.

How MMS works

Once the visible tumor has been removed (stage one), it is quartered and sliced horizontally. Each slice is analyzed under the microscope. From this, the surgeon can build up a "map" of the contours of the tumor (stage two).

Tissue is removed from targeted cancerous areas, sliced, and examined, and more cancerous cells are removed (stage three). The procedure continues until all cancerous cells have been removed (stage four).

Clinically evident cancer
Saucer-shaped excision
Remaining cancer cells
Bottom of surgical excision
Remaining cancer cells
All cancerous cells removed

Stage one   **Stage two**   **Stage three**   **Stage four**

HEALING AFTER MMS

Healing depends upon the size of the original tumor. Occasionally, the wound may be left to heal on its own. When very small growths (less than 1 inch) are excised, the edges of the wound will probably be stitched together. If stitches are used, they will be removed after 5 to 10 days, depending on the site. There will initially be a red scar, but this will gradually fade. It is important to protect the scar from further sun damage, and a sunblock should be used over it at all times to prevent it from overgrowing (a so-called hypertrophic scar).

When larger growths are removed, a skin graft may be taken from another part of the body—usually an area that is not seen, such as the buttock or thigh—to fill the gap. Dressings will be applied and checked regularly until the patient's own skin has has had time to grow over and fill the gap.

Occasionally, it may not be possible to fill the defect with a skin graft. In this case a plastic surgeon will create a skin flap—a small area of skin that is moved, along with its blood supply, from an area close to the wound site. Very good cosmetic results can be achieved with this technique, although this may not always be immediately apparent. It is important that patients ask their surgeon to show them photographs of previous surgeries for reassurance.

In the right hands, MMS is a highly effective method for treating basal cell and other carcinomas, and patients heal well. However, it should only be performed by doctors who have been specially trained and are experienced in the procedure.

Treating skin cancer

Although the majority of skin cancers are not fatal, they do cause disfiguring growths that can increase in size and destroy local structures in the skin. Early detection and management of such growths is extremely important.

Skin cancers can arise from any component of the skin, including the blood vessels, sweat glands, nerve fibers, fatty tissue, and muscle wall. However, all these skin cancers are relatively rare. For example, mycosis fungoides, which has an effect on the skin via the immune system, affects less than one in 10,000 people. By far the most common forms of skin cancer—basal cell carcinomas, squamous cell carcinomas, and malignant melanomas—arise from the epidermis of the skin.

SUN AND SKIN CANCER

There is increasing public awareness that one of the main causes of skin cancer is excess exposure to UV radiation from the sun, hence the tendency of cancerous growths to develop on parts of the body most often exposed to sunlight, such as the face, hands, and shoulders. People with very fair skin and those prone to sunburn are most at risk. Although it is true that incidences of skin cancer are higher in countries with lots of sunlight such as Australia and South Africa, it is important to remember that it is UV exposure that is the risk factor, and UV light can penetrate clouds.

BASAL CELL CARCINOMA (BCC)

The most common form of skin cancer is a basal cell carcinoma. It is sometimes referred to as a rodent ulcer because the growth does not spread elsewhere in the body but very slowly nibbles away at local tissue in a rodent-like manner. The outlook for a patient with a BCC is good because BBC does not spread to other areas of the body. If left untreated, however, a BCC can disfigure, so early recognition and treatment are important. There are about 1 million cases of BCCs each year in the U.S. alone.

There is no doubt that a major cause of BCCs is long-term exposure to sunlight. They are more frequently seen in patients over the age of 50, but now younger and younger people are developing such cancers, reflecting changes in attitudes and habits regarding sun exposure.

A rodent ulcer may first come to the patient's notice as a skin lesion or sore that fails to heal within a month or so or that bleeds spontaneously. It can be flesh-colored, pink, red, or brown like a mole. It can begin as a red patch or as a flat scarred area on the skin that may appear pale or white compared to the surrounding skin.

Treatment of a basal cell carcinoma

Management of these tumors depends to some extent on the type of tumor present, where it is located, its size, and the general health of the patient.

- **Curettage and cautery** This is the process of surgically removing the tumor by scraping away the surrounding tissue and then cauterizing the base as a way of both stopping bleeding and of destroying any tumor cells that may remain in the skin. This has a high cure rate and produces a very satisfactory cosmetic result.
- **Cryotherapy using liquid nitrogen** Freezing the BCC and thereby inducing a degree of cell damage and necrosis produces a good result for many patients, particularly

The effect of the sun on skin temperature
A thermogram uses photographic film sensitive to UV radiation to measure the heat given off by various parts of the body. The man's face starts off cool (yellow to green, 86–90°F, top left) but soon becomes much hotter (red, 95°F, bottom right).

a This red ulcerlike growth is a basal cell carcinoma on the face. It started as a small, flat nodule and then slowly broke down in the center to form a shallow ulcer.
b Here it is being treated by radiation. The patient has lead blocks (covered with plastic wrap) on her eye and cheek to protect healthy cells from the radiation. The machine focuses X-rays that slow or stop the growth of abnormal cells on the BCC.
c Three months after radiation treatment, the BCC is gone and only a pink patch remains.

can initially look fairly acceptable, but years later there may be some significant appearance of scar tissue and broken blood vessels at the site of treatment.

- **Topical therapy** The use of a cream such as 5 Flurouracil can produce a good cure for BCCs, especially those on the lower legs, where surgery or radiation would not be advisable because these areas can heal poorly.
- **Photodynamic therapy** Many treatment centers have reported good results with this treatment. The combined use of a cream and light source produces cell destruction at the tumor site (see page 111). The cosmetic results can be excellent. Evidence to date suggests that the risk of recurrence is similar to that of other treatments, although long-term data has yet to be published.
- **Mohs micrographic surgery** has been around for many years (see page 128).

What are the chances of a second BCC?

It has been estimated that 40 percent of patients will develop a new BCC within 5 years of the first. With this in mind, anyone who has developed a BCC should do what he or she can to reduce the chances of this happening by limiting sun exposure, wearing adequate protection when in the sun and checking skin on a regular basis for any suspicious lesions.

SQUAMOUS CELL CARCINOMA (SCC)

The second most common type of skin cancer in the U.S. is a squamous cell carcinoma. An SCC often takes the form of a lump, which may ulcerate, become crusty and bleed, and be quite painful to touch. There is a small risk of such a tumor spreading to another part of the body. It is estimated that about 1.2 million SCCs are diagnosed every year in the U.S., and the number is increasing.

The development of a squamous cell carcinoma is usually related to chronic UV exposure, much like BCCs, and therefore SCCs too are especially common on the sun-damaged skin of fair-skinned people. Alternatively, an SCC may develop as a result of previous exposure to radiation, in a patient who has a chronic wound in the skin, or in a patient who has impaired immune function.

Treatment of a squamous cell carcinoma

The main aims of treatment are the destruction of the primary growth and the prevention of the tumor spreading elsewhere. The earlier the diagnosis and treatment, the better.

those with growths on the back. A disadvantage is that the freezing often produces a wound that can take from a few weeks to a few months to heal fully.

- **Ablative laser therapy** For patients with a number of BCCs on their trunk and back, a carbon dioxide laser can be an effective, rapid treatment. It removes tissue and keeps bleeding to a minimum. Unfortunately, there is as yet little data on this therapy's long-term effectiveness.
- **Excision of the actual growth** The growth on the skin is cut out and then the defect is closed up with sutures. Alternatively, a flap made of local skin may be used (see page 121) or a skin graft if the defect is very large.
- **Radiation** Many dermatology centers now have combined clinics where a dermatologist, radiologist, and surgeon decide together on the best treatment for each patient. For some patients, the demands of frequent attendance at the center for radiation sessions can be a problem. There is also the disadvantage that scarring

REMOVAL OF A MALIGNANT MELANOMA

I only mentioned to my doctor in passing the appearance of a small dark mole on my tummy. He booked me into a dermatologist office "just in case."

After examining the mole, the dermatologist said she wanted to remove the mole that very afternoon. The operation began with a local anesthetic by injection, then the doctor *made two curved incisions into the skin on either side of the mole. The mole was taken out, and the cut was secured with a few stitches. The whole procedure was completely painless.*

The mole was sent off for biopsy. A week later I received the bad news that it was a malignant melanoma. I returned to the office the next day,

when more of the area around the mole was cut away—again under local anesthetic. Since then there has been no sign of the cancer spreading. I have been very lucky.

- **Surgical excision** is the treatment of choice, depending on the patient's age and health and the site of the tumor.
- **Curettage and cautery** can produce a very good result.
- **Radiation** can be effective.
- **Mohs micrographic surgery** has been used for the management of squamous cell carcinomas.

Treatment is followed up with regular skin surveillance and advice to the patient on adequate sun protection.

MALIGNANT MELANOMA

The most worrisome type of skin malignancy is a malignant melanoma. About 54,000 melanomas are diagnosed in the United States every year.

A malignant melanoma can occur spontaneously or can develop from a preexisting mole. In terms of the risk of developing a malignant melanoma, it is not so much chronic ultraviolet exposure as periods of sunburn, particularly in childhood, that appear to be important.

Occasionally, a malignant melanoma develops from a mole that was present at birth (the vast majority of moles appear during childhood and adolescence).

Treatment of a malignant melanoma

As with other skin cancers, the aim is early detection and early management. Any change in a mole's condition (see page 107) should be reported to the physician immediately.

- **Surgery** The principle treatment for malignant melanoma remains surgical intervention. The mole is removed with a safety margin of skin around the mole to ensure, as far as possible, that all the cancerous cells have been removed.
- **Regular monitoring** After the mole has been removed, a patient is given a full skin check at regular intervals to be sure that the growth has not reappeared in the scar itself or anywhere else. These checks take place for at least 5 years after the operation. In addition, patients are taught how to examine their own skin thoroughly so they can look out for suspicious growths.

In recent years, patients and doctors have been picking up more malignant melanomas much earlier than before, which leads to a better outcome for more patients.

If a malignant melanoma recurs, further surgery, chemotherapy, radiation, and vaccination therapy (the injection of antigens to stimulate the immune system to fight the cancer cells) are all possibilities.

Squamous carcinoma cells
An immunofluorescent light micrograph shows squamous carcinoma cells cultured from a tumor.

A TO Z

OF DISEASES AND DISORDERS

This section gives information on the main illnesses and medical conditions that can affect the skin, hair, and nails.

This index is arranged alphabetically, and each entry is structured in a similar way:

What are the causes?

What are the symptoms?

How is it diagnosed?

What are the treatment options?

What is the outlook?

ACNE

A condition in which excess sebum and a growth change in cells in the hair follicle leads to blockage of skin pores. These can become inflamed and infected, appearing as spots on the skin.

What are the causes?

This very common condition is a disorder of the hair follicles and associated sebaceous glands, which produce sebum. Excess production is triggered by hormonal changes at puberty, and there may be a family history of acne.

What are the symptoms?

A variety of skin lesions are seen—ranging from noninflamed blackheads and whiteheads, to inflamed papules and pustules, to large nodular lesions and cysts. The larger lesions may leave scarring once healed.

Acne commonly affects the face, back, shoulders, and chest and ranges in severity from mild to severe. It can be a distressing condition for the self-conscious teenager and also in adults who feel they should have grown out of it.

What are the treatment options?

In mild acne, creams or lotions applied directly to the affected areas (known as "topical" treatments) may be sufficient. These preparations can be antibiotic agents that unblock skin pores, or a combination of the two.

DEFINITIONS

BIOPSY Removal of a piece of skin under local anesthetic for diagnostic purposes.

ERYTHEMA Used in dermatology to mean redness of the skin.

EXCORIATIONS Breaks in the skin surface caused by scratching.

LESION General term used to indicate any abnormality of the skin.

MACULE A flat area of altered skin.

NODULE A large papule.

PAPULE Small raised bump on the skin surface.

PATCH Flat area of affected skin, larger than a macule.

PLAQUE A patch that is raised above the surface level of the skin.

PUSTULE A papule containing pus.

SEBUM Oily substance produced by sebaceous glands within the skin.

In more serious cases, tablet treatments are used. Females can use a particular form of the oral contraceptive pill, which helps because of its hormonal action. In both males and females, antibiotics are helpful when used regularly for at least 6 months. These should be used in combination with a topical vitamin A drug to unblock the pores.

For severe acne, isotretinoin is a treatment option. This is a course of tablets for at least 4 months and is available by prescription from dermatologists. Blood tests are required before and during treatment, and because fetal abnormalities can result from taking this drug, effective contraception must be in place before it starts. The drug has been implicated in depression and suicide attempts, and this risk must be made known to the patient and parents. Phototherapy (p. 112) can help, and larger cysts may be treated with steroid injections.

No matter what the severity, regular gentle cleansing of the face is recommended. It is unlikely that any change in diet will improve the condition.

The majority of people will be clear of acne by their mid 20s, but it can persist to the 30s, 40s, and beyond.

ACTINIC (SOLAR) KERATOSES

These can be premalignant lesions, not cancerous in themselves, but they may become so if left untreated.

What are the causes?

As the name suggests, this condition arises from excess sun exposure with inadequate protection.

What are the symptoms?

These lesions may be present singly or in large numbers and are most common in the fair-skinned. Men are affected more frequently than women. They appear as warty papules or patches with a rough, scaly surface. They may be pink, gray, or brown and are usually asymptomatic. The face, scalp, ears, and back of hands are most commonly affected.

How is it diagnosed?

They are generally diagnosed on appearance, but a biopsy can be performed if necessary.

What are the treatment options?

Anyone with solar keratoses should cover up in the sun and use a sunscreen on any exposed areas of skin.

Individual lesions can be treated with cryotherapy (p. 119), but if large areas are affected, particularly on the face, this may not be practical. Regular application of a topical chemotherapy cream for 4 weeks may eradicate them over 2 to 3 months. Particularly stubborn lesions or those with doubtful diagnosis can be removed under local anesthetic.

What is the outlook?
There is a small risk that keratoses can become cancerous, so any areas that are changing or not responding to treatment should be reported to your doctor. Also, people affected by solar keratoses are at an increased risk of other sun-related skin cancers and should get new or suspicious areas checked by their doctor as soon as possible.

ALBINISM
A condition characterized by hereditary lack of pigment.

What are the causes?
Albinism is a genetically transmitted condition occurring in roughly 1 in 17,000 people in the United States. A defect in pigment production leads to white or pink skin, blond or white hair, and lack of color in the eyes. Those affected tolerate sun poorly because they burn easily, and they often have poor eyesight.

How is it diagnosed?
Diagnosis can be made in the uterus with fetal skin biopsy, and this may be advised in tropical countries. After birth, the diagnosis is apparent without investigation.

What are the treatment options?
The main treatment is sun avoidance through regular use of at least a SPF 50 sunblock and sun-protective clothing.

What is the outlook?
A small amount of pigment may appear with age. In temperate climates, the prognosis is good: People with albinism can live relatively normally. In the tropics, early development of skin cancers makes the outlook worse.

ALOPECIA AREATA
Loss of hair in discrete coin-shaped areas.

What are the causes?
This is thought to be caused by an exaggerated immune response targeted at the hair root. There may be a background of affected family members, and in some cases it seems to follow emotional or physical trauma.

What are the symptoms?
Rounded patches of hair loss occur, with a distinct edge and normal skin on the exposed scalp. It usually starts to appear in the teens and 20s. Hair can be taken for analysis or a biopsy taken if there is any doubt of the diagnosis.

What are the treatment options?
If the patch is fairly small and causes no concern, no treatment is needed. For larger areas, steroids can be used either as a lotion or injected into the affected skin. Phototherapy may be helpful in severe cases. In 70 to 80 percent of cases, hair regrowth—usually white—occurs without treatment, although recurrent episodes are not unusual. A small percentage may progress to total hair loss.

BASAL CELL CARCINOMA (BCC)
The most common form of skin cancer.

What are the causes?
BCC affects males more often than females, especially on the face. Like many skin cancers, it is most commonly caused by sun exposure over many years. It is thought that excess sun up to the age of 20 is the most important factor, although BCCs generally do not develop until middle age or later.

What are the symptoms?
There are different types of BCCs. The most common tends to start as a slow-growing nodule with a pearly edge containing visible blood vessels. As it grows—which is a slow process—it tends to ulcerate in the middle—hence the alternative name "rodent ulcer." ("Rodent" because if left alone it eats away slowly at the surrounding skin and tissues.) The next most common type is a red scaly plaque that slowly increases in size. It lies more superficially in the skin, hence the name superficial BCC. In a third type, morpheaform BCC, the cancer cells induce a reaction in the skin with the production of almost a scar. The skin feels firm and may have blood vessels on the surface.

The appearance suggests the diagnosis, which is confirmed by biopsy.

What are the treatment options?
Removal under local anesthetic is the likely treatment. Freezing with liquid nitrogen is sometimes successful for superficial tumors, and photodynamic therapy is becoming common (p. 111).

What is the outlook?
The outlook for BCC is very good because it does not spread to other areas of the body. Having had one nodule increases the risk of developing more, so regular checkups and avoidance of excess sun are essential.

BIRTHMARKS
Common skin markings that vary in severity from minor to disfiguring—not all are present from birth.

CAPILLARY HEMANGIOMA
Also known as strawberry nevis, these appear in the first four weeks of life as a tiny red spot and grow over a few weeks to produce a deep red swelling composed of blood vessels, with a soft, spongy feel. One in five infants have more than one. These resolve with age—50 percent are gone within five years and 75 percent within seven years. If they affect vision or feeding or bleed excessively, systemic steroids, surgery, or laser treatment may be needed.

CONGENITAL MELANOCYTIC NEVUS (MOLE)
Ten percent of the population are born with one or more moles. These start as flat circular or oval areas of pigmentation but often change in appearance at puberty. They may become raised or slightly warty. Normal moles have an even color and even border. Large moles or those sited in awkward places can be removed. See Moles (pp. 147–148).

EPIDERMAL NEVUS
Present from birth or developing later in adulthood, this has a warty or velvety appearance. They can be removed by cryotherapy (p. 119) or laser therapy (pp. 126–27).

MONGOLIAN SPOT
A bluish-black birthmark on the lower back, most common in Asian and African races, which clears in later childhood.

NEVUS FLAMMEUS
Also known as port wine stains, these darker red or purplish patches are seen on the face or upper body. They tend to affect one side of the body and do not cross the midline. Those around the eye may extend internally and can cause epilepsy. They do not resolve without treatment but can respond to laser treatment or be covered with cosmetics.

NEVUS SEBACEOUS
A hairless red or orange plaque on the scalp, which may grow and become warty at puberty. Skin cancer can develop in these birthmarks, so they should be monitored or removed.

SALMON PATCH
Also known as stork marks, these pinkish-red patches on the forehead or back of the neck are very common. Salmon patches on the forehead usually resolve over a few years; those on the neck tend to remain into adulthood.

BLISTERS
Blisters are caused by an accumulation of fluid within the top layers of the skin.

Small blisters are known as "vesicles," larger ones as "bullae." There are a number of causes of blistering disorders including infection (chicken pox and shingles, for example), dermatitis, trauma, bites, sunburn, medicines, and autoimmune diseases such as pemphigoid/pemphigus (pp. 149–150). Treatment depends on the underlying cause.

BOILS
A boil is tender, red skin nodule caused by infection of a hair follicle with Staphylococcus bacteria.

After about a week, pus is visible under the skin; this can be painful and swollen until the boil bursts and the pus drains. Keeping the area clean and applying warm compresses several times a day to bring the boil to a head are usually all that is required. Large painful boils, however, can be lanced by a doctor. Occasionally, antibiotics can limit the spread of infection. A furuncle is another term for boil; a collection of boils is a carbuncle.

BOWEN'S DISEASE
A precancerous condition that progresses slowly.

What are the causes?
Bowen's disease can be caused by excess sun exposure and has been linked to arsenic ingestion. Cancerous cells may be seen under microscopic examination. They are confined to the surface of the skin and are generally easily treated.

What are the symptoms?

Typically, Bowen's disease is found on the shins of middle-aged or elderly women, although men may be affected. It may also be seen elsewhere on the body. It appears as a dark pink scaly patch with a distinct edge but generally does not cause any other symptoms. It may take years to become an inch in diameter.

What are the treatment options?

If the patch is small, it can be removed under local anesthetic. However, cryotherapy (p. 119) is often sufficient. Photodynamic therapy (p. 111) is increasingly being used. Your doctor may also prescribe treatment in a cream form (5-fluorouracil). Although very slow growing if left untreated, Bowen's disease does have the potential to develop into squamous cell carcinoma (p. 154), so treatment is required once it has been detected.

CELLULITIS
An acute bacterial infection of the skin.

Although cellulitis can happen to anyone, it develops more often in diabetics or those with poor circulation. In this condition, skin becomes red, hot, swollen, and tender, often with painful enlargement of nearby lymph nodes. There may be an obvious entry for the infection such as a bite or cut. Antibiotics are used to clear the infection, either orally or intravenously depending on the severity. Some individuals may have recurrent episodes.

Necrotizing fasciitis is a particularly aggressive type of cellulitis in which the affected area becomes dusky, blistered, and numb. If left untreated, the affected skin and underlying tissue eventually die off.

CHERRY ANGIOMA
These common skin lesions are caused by an overgrowth of small blood vessels in the skin.

These lesions appear as bright red papules, particularly on the trunk in the middle-aged and elderly. No treatment is necessary because the condition is benign.

CHICKEN POX
A viral infection that is common, particularly in children, and is caused by infection with the varicella zoster virus, a type of herpes virus.

What are the symptoms?

The rash consists of small blisters that burst and crust over and may heal to leave small white scars. It is itchy, and the whole body may be affected. It may be preceded by cold symptoms. Diagnosis is made on appearance.

What are the treatment options?

Generally, no treatment is needed. Bathing and the use of calamine lotion can help relieve the itch. Chicken pox is contagious until the spots dry (and for several days before they appear). The incubation period is about 14 days. Chicken pox is rarely caught more than once, although shingles may develop years after chicken pox infection. Pregnant women who have not previously had chicken pox should contact their doctor if exposed, because there is a risk to the unborn baby and vaccination may be required.

CHILBLAINS (PERNIOSIS)
Purple-pink swellings particularly on the fingers, toes, and ears that result from exposure to cold weather.

Chilblains are a common condition caused by exaggerated "shut down" of blood vessels in response to cold. They are more common in females and the elderly—possibly because they do not wrap up well enough in cold weather—and can be painful and itchy. Symptoms tend to be worse when warming up after exposure to the cold. Avoidance of cold is the main treatment. Weak steroid creams or medicines that open up the blood vessels may help. Chilblains settle in time, but recurrences are common.

CHONDRODERMATITIS NODULARIS HELICIS (CNH)
Painful nodules on the outer ear caused by inflammation of the cartilage.

The trigger for this painful condition, which may cause sleep disturbance if the nodules are rolled on during the night, is probably pressure on the ear during sleep. They are diagnosed on appearance. Treatment is usually in the form of removal under local anesthetic, although cryotherapy (p. 119) may be used. The condition may recur, in which case a protective mold can be made to relieve pressure on the nodule, thereby avoiding further surgery.

CONTACT DERMATITIS
An allergic or irritant reaction to one or more environmental triggers.

What are the causes?
The condition is caused by external substances contacting the skin and causing eczema. The substances may be irritants (which would cause a similar reaction in anyone with ongoing exposure to the irritant) or allergens (which cause an allergic reaction only in susceptible individuals). In addition, irritant reactions tend to be gradual in onset, whereas allergic reactions are more immediate. Nickel is the most common cause of skin allergy, but glues, leathers, dyes, cosmetics, creams, chemicals, and detergents may all cause irritant reactions.

What are the symptoms?
The hands and face are commonly involved, but the site will depend on the area of the body that is in contact with the trigger. Nickel, found in a wide range of jewelry and other products, may cause a reaction on the ears or neck or other areas where the skin is exposed: Studs in clothing, for example, can affect the lower abdomen. Some allergies are only activated when exposed to sunlight, a phenomenon known as photodermatitis.

The structure of stainless steel is such that the nickel it contains does not leach out onto the skin, so people with contact dermatitis can wear stainless steel jewelry or watch straps.

How is it diagnosed?
Individuals will often recognize a trigger at work or at home. However, patch testing is sometimes used to identify the cause of allergic dermatitis. This involves application of small amounts of common allergens to the back for 48 hours (pp. 109–110) and then removing and looking for any reaction two days later.

What are the treatment options?
The main treatment is avoidance of identified irritants or allergens. Protective clothing may be necessary (for mechanics with hand-contact dermatitis, for example). Treatment is the same as for eczema. If known allergens or irritants can be avoided, the skin should settle.

CYST
A fluid-filled "walled" lesion deep within the dermis.

It is still unclear why cysts appear. Some babies are born with one or more, there may be a family history of the problem, and they are more likely in smokers. Small cysts do not need treatment, but larger ones should be removed. Removal involves cutting out the whole cyst, including the wall, and then stitching the wound. Cysts can, however, recur. If a cyst becomes infected, antibiotics may be necessary.

DERMATITIS ARTEFACTA
These are self-inflicted skin lesions.

The lesions are often bizarre in both shape and appearance and tend to be found on accessible areas. Teenage girls and young women are often affected, and there may be other evidence of psychological distress. Sufferers generally deny having any part in the condition, and doctors base a diagnosis on clinical judgement (a biopsy may be performed to exclude a genuine skin condition). The lesions are difficult to treat until the underlying psychological condition improves. It is important for the doctor to maintain sympathetic contact and to avoid confronting and alienating the patient. Psychotherapy or psychiatric referral may be indicated because the condition may last for years.

DERMATITIS HERPETIFORMIS
A very itchy skin disease associated with celiac disease affecting males more often than females.

The cause of this disease is unclear. It is found with celiac disease (inability to absorb gluten from the intestine), although the sufferer may be unaware of any bowel problem when consulting the doctor about the rash. Small intensely itchy blisters are found on the elbows, knees, neck, shoulder, and back, and a biopsy is required to confirm the diagnosis. Dapsone tablets may be prescribed initially to control symptoms, but those affected should see a gastroenterologist for investigation into associated bowel problems, and a gluten-free diet should be commenced. Improvement is often rapid once treatment is started. The disease is controlled by a gluten-free diet, dapsone, or both.

DERMATOFIBROMA
Benign nodules immediately under the skin surface.

This common condition is thought to be a local reaction to some form of injury, such as an insect bite, although the initial event may not be remembered. Dermatofibromas appear as firm nodules that usually cause no symptoms. They may be skin-colored but are often darker. They are found most commonly in young women, particularly on the lower legs. A biopsy will be helpful to rule out anything more serious if the diagnosis is unclear. Irritating nodules can be removed under local anesthetic, but because they are benign, no treatment may be necessary.

DIAPER RASH
A raw, often blistering rash on a baby's skin.

What are the causes?
The most common cause of diaper rash is irritation from prolonged contact with urine and feces, although the occurrence of diaper rash is falling because of the increased use of absorbent disposable diapers. Diaper rash can also be caused by infection with candida (the organism which causes thrush) and may be one of the areas affected by seborrheic dermatitis (p. 153). Psoriasis is a rare cause of diaper rash, as is eczema.

What are the symptoms?
The skin becomes red, inflamed, and sore, and there may be blistering and ulceration in more severe cases. In simple cases of irritant diaper rash, the skin folds in the groin tend to be spared but are involved in candidal and seborrheic cases. In candidal diaper rash, small satellite spots may be seen separate from the main area of redness.

What are the treatment options?
Diapers should be changed frequently. At each change, the diaper area should be cleaned thoroughly with a soap substitute or simply water. Liberal amounts of diaper cream, such as petroleum jelly, should then be applied. Baby wipes may contain fragrance that can irritate broken skin, so these should not be used. Diapers should be left off for short periods. In candidal infection or seborrheic dermatitis, a steroid cream combined with an antifungal agent may help.

ECZEMA
Eczema and dermatitis are synonymous. The condition involves acute or subacute inflammation of the skin centered in the epidermis and upper dermis.

Eczemas can be divided into exogenous (those caused by external factors) and endogenous (those related to a constitutional tendency to developing the eczema). The exogenous eczemas are contact irritant and contact allergic dermatitis (p. 138). The endogenous eczemas are atopic eczema, nummular eczema, and pompholyx.

ATOPIC ECZEMA
Atopic eczema is the most common eczema in childhood, affecting about 10 percent of children in the United States. In the vast majority of patients, it starts in childhood. Most do not have the condition as adults, but a few do have eczema through to adult life. Reactivation in adult life is often associated with work and is most common in people who have to wash their skin frequently, such as nurses, car mechanics, and hairdressers. In infancy, the eczema often affects the face, but in childhood it usually affects the skin creases in front of the elbows and behind the knees. In adult life, it focuses again on the face and also on the hands.

The problem with the skin is threefold:
- The skin is dry and dry skin is irritable.
- Where the eczema develops, the inflammation leads to further irritation.
- Scratching of irritated skin leads to loss of barrier function and allows infection to get in. Infection, particularly with *Staphylococcus aureus*, leads to worsening of the eczema not only at the site that is infected but also at distant sites.

Atopic eczema is associated with asthma and hay fever, and there is often a family history of asthma, eczema, or hay fever. Treatment is with daily baths, avoidance of detergents, use of emollients to wash the skin, copious moisturizers and appropriate strengths of topical corticosteroids, and topical or systemic antibiotics to treat infection.

Contact between patients with atopic eczema and those with cold sores must be avoided: the virus that causes cold sores can cause a widespread infection in the atopic individual that can spread to the blood and the brain.

NUMMULAR ECZEMA
This very aggressive eczema occurs usually in later life, in the 50s and 60s. The areas of eczema are round or coin shaped, well-demarcated red areas that have a rough surface and are extremely itchy. Secondary infection is common. The disease is self-limiting and usually lasts for about 18 months. Treatment involves the use of emollients and moisturizers and relatively strong topical corticosteroids with antibiotics topically or systemically when infection occurs.

POMPHOLYX

Pompholyx is an acute or subacute eczema affecting the hands (cheiro-pompholyx) or the feet (pedo-pompholyx). Because the skin in these areas is very thick, the inflammation leads to accumulation of small collections of fluid, allowing little vesicles—which look rather like sago grains in the skin—to develop. In the acute phase the skin is very itchy, but as it goes through to a subacute and chronic phase, the skin becomes thicker and drier, so that fissures and splits can occur on the fingers and palms. Special care should be exercised in looking after the skin of affected areas. Affected persons should avoid contact with detergents, wearing rubber gloves for wet work, but for no longer than 15 minutes at a time because this leads to sweating and softening of the skin. Rubber gloves should even be worn when washing hair because shampoo contains high levels of detergent. Copious amounts of moisturizer and emollients should be used, and strong topical corticosteroids are normally needed to control the disease. Secondary infection does occur and needs to be treated with antibiotics.

ERYTHEMA MULTIFORME
A toxic skin eruption triggered by several factors.

What are the causes?
The most common cause is herpes simplex infection (the virus that causes cold sores and genital herpes). Other viruses may be responsible, as can bacterial and fungal infections, drugs, pregnancy, and malignant disease. In 50 percent of cases, no cause is identified.

What are the symptoms?
The typical pattern is eruption of red, circular, nonscaly plaques that clear from the center to give typical "target" lesions. The hands and feet are most commonly affected, but this condition can also occur in the mucous lining of the mouth and the eyes, a condition known as Steven Johnson syndrome. A severe variant exists in which the top layer of the skin is shed (known as toxic epidermal necrolysis). A biopsy can confirm the diagnosis.

What are the treatment options?
Identification and removal of the underlying cause is the mainstay of treatment. If large areas are affected, oral steroids or hospital admission may be required. Individual lesions last a few days and several appear over 1 to 2 weeks until the underlying cause is removed.

ERYTHEMA NODOSUM
An inflammation of the subcutaneous fat.

This condition mostly affects young women and may be caused by a variety of infections or drug treatments. It may also indicate an underlying disease. In some cases, no cause is found. Painful, dusky-red nodules a half inch to 2 inches in diameter, are seen typically on the shins, sometimes with associated joint pains. Physical examination, chest X-rays, and blood testing will help identify an underlying cause, and a biopsy can be taken. Rest and antiinflammatory drugs will relieve the pain. Any underlying cause should be treated. Individual lesions clear up in 6 to 8 weeks, but the condition may persist if the cause is not found and removed.

FISH TANK GRANULOMA
A condition found in people who are involved in cleaning tropical fish tanks.

This condition is caused by a mycobacterium that lives in fish tanks. It enters the skin through tiny breaks when the hands are in the water. These result in reddish-blue nodules, either singly or in groups, on the hands and forearms. The diagnosis is made on the appearance of the skin, and a biopsy can confirm this. Sick fish must be removed from the tank, and gloves should be worn when cleaning it. Antibiotics can be used, as can steroid creams, but often not putting bare hands in tank water is all that is necessary. Even after successful treatment, it may take months or years for the nodules to clear up.

FOLLICULITIS
Infection or inflammation of one or more hair follicles caused by bacterial or yeast infection.

Folliculitis is more common in overweight people and diabetics, and it may be triggered by hair removal (by waxing or shaving, for example). Pustules appear in hair-bearing areas, often the beard area in men and legs in women.

Furuncles and carbuncles are related conditions where one or more hair follicles are infected, forming an abscess.

What are the treatment options?
A microbiological swab can be taken to confirm the presence of infection and indicate the most appropriate treatment. Oral antibiotics and antibiotic cream are used to treat bacterial folliculitis. Yeast folliculitis responds to antifungal drugs. Folliculitis may be recurrent, in which case the use

of antiseptic washes in the bath or shower can help keep infection at bay. Carbuncles may need to be drained.

FUNGAL INFECTIONS (RINGWORM)
These extremely common skin infections can affect several parts of the body.

Fungal infection can be contracted from other people or animals and can affect the skin, hair, and nails.

What are the symptoms?
These depend on the type and site of the infection. The most common type of ringworm (or tinea) is tinea pedis (athlete's foot), which appears as scaly or soggy skin between the toes, especially the fourth and fifth toes. There may also be dry scaly skin on the feet with blistering.

Any area of skin can be involved in ringworm, with the rash appearing as red patches with a distinct, scaly edge (the "ring") which is often itchy. Toenails are affected more commonly than fingernails. They become yellow, crumbly, and thickened and may separate from the nail bed.

Ringworm affects the scalp in children more than adults, with scaly, coin-shaped areas of hair loss and scaly or clogged inflamed swelling with overlying hair loss (a kerion).

How is it diagnosed?
Diagnosis should be confirmed, particularly in nail infection, before treatment is started. Skin scrapings, nail clippings, or hair pluckings are taken and sent for analysis.

What are the treatment options?
Antifungal creams are sufficient to clear up most skin infections, but if extensive, a course of oral treatment may be required. Antifungal nail lacquers are effective in some nail infections, but more commonly a 6- to 12-week course of tablets is needed. Scalp infection requires oral treatment. Treatment is generally effective, but recurrence is common.

Steroids should be avoided: They cause the rash to worsen and may change its appearance, making diagnosis difficult.

GRANULOMA ANNULARE
Lesions most commonly found on the hands and feet, although they can be more widespread.

The cause is not known, although widespread cases of granuloma annulare can be associated with diabetes. It commonly affects children and young adults and is more often seen in females.

What are the symptoms?
The typical lesion consists of a clear center surrounded by a collection of nodules forming a circle roughly 1 inch in diameter. The nodules may be purple or skin-colored.

What are the treatment options?
There is no truly effective treatment, but steroid creams or steroid injection into the affected area may be used. A urine sample should be tested for glucose to check for diabetes. Granuloma annulare resolves without treatment over several months to years, although recurrences are common.

HAIR LOSS
A common condition in both men and women, often known as alopecia.

What are the causes?
Generalized hair loss or thinning can have a variety of causes. The most common is androgenic alopecia, or male-pattern baldness, which can affect men from the teens. Half of women 50 or over are also affected to some extent, and the number increases with age in both sexes.

Abnormalities of the thyroid or pituitary glands, dietary deficiencies (p. 71), and certain medication, notably in chemotherapy, can lead to hair loss, which should be reversible with treatment or removing the underlying cause.

Another cause is a condition known as telogen effluvium, in which a large number of hairs are shed simultaneously, often about three months after an episode of physical or psychological stress (such as childbirth). This condition requires no treatment and normality returns in time.

What are the treatment options?
Most people with thinning hair require no treatment, and indeed, treatment can be quite unsatisfactory. Lotions are available to apply to the scalp, and many patients derive some benefit from tablets. Private surgery in the form of hair transplant may be an option, and wigs can be prescribed by a hospital specialist.

Androgenic alopecia is progressive, although the degree of hair loss varies from one individual to another. If there is an underlying cause, hair loss is usually reversed when the cause is dealt with.

HEAD LICE
Infection with head lice is common, especially in primary school children, but any age can be affected.

What are the causes?
Head lice are not related to hygiene: They infect clean and dirty hair alike. The head louse cannot jump or fly and spreads between people by walking across hair, so only close head-to-head contacts can be infected.

What are the symptoms?
Itching of the scalp or neck is the main symptom, and red spots are seen that may become infected with scabbing. Lice may be seen on the scalp. Empty egg cases are often seen attached to the base of hairs. These do not indicate active infection. Insecticidal treatment is only recommended if live lice are present. The easiest way to check for live lice is by combing through sections of wet, conditioned hair. Wiping the comb on a tissue will reveal any lice present.

What are the treatment options?
A variety of preparations can be bought from the pharmacist, but it is best to avoid alcohol-based treatments, which are highly flammable and can be irritants and trigger an asthma attack in susceptible individuals.

Head lice live for 30 days on the head but only 24 hours off it. The female lays up to 100 eggs, which take 7 to 10 days to hatch; 10 days later a female can begin to lay eggs.

The preparation should be applied to clean, dry hair before going to bed, left to dry naturally, and washed out the next morning. This should be repeated after 7 days. Empty egg cases are not removed by this treatment, and have to be physically removed by combing. An alternative treatment is the "bug-busting" approach (p. 59). Kits are available from pharmacists, and the treatment involves combing wet, conditioned hair every 3 days for at least 2 weeks.

Failure to check and treat close contacts is a common cause of reinfection. Two to 3 days after the second treatment, detection combing should be repeated. If treatment hasn't been successful, make an appointment with your doctor or the school nurse for more advice.

HERPES SIMPLEX
The herpes simplex virus causes cold sores on the body and the genitals.

The condition consists of painful blisters, which can ulcerate and clear after 7 to 10 days. Attacks may be recurrent and are contagious. Cold sores can be treated early with antiviral cream, which should be applied as soon as tingling is felt and before the blisters appear. Genital herpes can be treated with antiviral tablets, and condoms should be used to protect sexual partners from infection.

HIDRADENITIS SUPPURATIVA
Hidradenitis is a fairly common disorder of the apocrine glands of the skin.

What are the symptoms?
The condition starts usually between ages 20 and 30 and is more common in females. Painful, inflamed nodules and abscesses are seen in the groin, armpits, and sometimes the neck, often with blackheads that may leave scarring. Sufferers have 4 to 5 new boils a month in typical sites, each of which may be sore for about 7 days. Stress, heat, sweating, and friction tend to make it worse, and it is more common in smokers.

What are the treatment options?
Antiseptic washes and antibiotic creams may be enough in mild cases, but often long-term courses of antibiotics (lasting at least 3 months) are necessary. In women, a type of contraceptive pill can be useful.

In severe cases with multiple lesions, steroid tablets may be used for a few days, and isotretinoin—available by prescription from dermatologists—can also help. It is an effective treatment but can cause fetal abnormalities if taken in pregnancy, so precautions must be taken before initiating this treatment. Surgery can be used for acute abscesses.

What is the outlook?
Hidradenitis often runs a prolonged course and may be present for up to 20 years after diagnosis. It may disappear in women after menopause, because of hormonal changes.

HIRSUTISM
Hirsutism describes the growth of hair in a male pattern on the body and face of a female.

What are the causes?
In most cases, no cause is found, and it is simply caused by an increased sensitivity to male hormones that are normally found in the female circulation. Polycystic ovarian syndrome is a known cause, and abnormalities of the pituitary or adrenal glands are less common causes.

What are the symptoms?

Excess hair is seen mainly down the midline of the body—lips, chin, sternum, and abdomen. Menstrual irregularities may be present, and the skin may be greasy. A blood test can confirm an underlying ovarian or gland problem, and polycystic ovaries will be visible on an ultrasound scan.

What are the treatment options?

Any underlying medical condition should be treated. Bleaching can be tried, as can hair removal by plucking or shaving. A beautician can advise on waxing or electrolysis, and laser hair removal is available in some hospitals. A form of the oral contraceptive pill is used in polycystic ovarian syndrome to counteract the male hormones and to regularize periods. Patients who are overweight often benefit from a weight loss program.

In cases where no cause is found, symptoms tend to start at puberty and may worsen with age.

HYPERHIDROSIS

Hyperhidrosis is an excess production of sweat.

What are the causes?

Excess sweat production may be localized in the palms, soles, and armpits or generalized over the whole body. It may be caused by heat, emotion, medicines, shock, or a disorder of the glands or nerves controlling sweating. Generalized increased sweating is more likely if an underlying cause is present; blood tests or X-rays may be performed if an underlying condition is suspected.

What are the treatment options?

Aluminium chloride-based antiperspirant lotions can be applied in affected areas—these are available from a doctor and may be all that is required.

For stubborn cases, a process called iontophoresis can be performed in hospitals. This involves the passage of a low voltage electrical current across the skin. Several treatments are required, and the course may need to be repeated or continued to keep symptoms under control.

Surgery is required in some cases to interrupt the nerves which supply the sweat glands. A new approach is the use of Botox® injections into the affected areas of skin.

ICHTHYOSIS

A condition resulting in a scalelike appearance of the skin; the term is derived from the Greek for "fish."

What are the causes?

A combination of increased production of skin cells and altered adhesion between cells causes dead cells or "scales" to remain stuck to the skin surface. Ichthyosis may be inherited, although the condition can develop later in life.

What are the symptoms?

The most common form of ichthyosis, ichthyosis vulgaris, affects 1 person in 300 and first appears in infancy. Persistent mild scaling of the back, abdomen, thighs, and upper arms is seen, which worsens in winter. Another form, recessive ichthyosis, is carried on the X chromosome and affects males only, causing large, dark scales on the neck, buttocks, trunk, and limbs. Female carriers of the condition can suffer prolonged labor because of the lack of the enzyme steroid sulfatase. The condition does not tend to improve with age. More severe inherited forms exist; they are generally evident from birth.

The development of acquired ichthyosis later in life is unusual and may indicate underlying illness. It is important to differentiate between this and normal drying of the skin later in life.

What are the treatment options?

Emollients, both as soap substitutes and moisturizers, are the mainstay of treatment and are combined with gentle abrasion to remove the scales. Creams containing weak concentrations of salicylic acid can dissolve the scales, but care must be taken on broken skin and in infants, as absorption can lead to internal organ damage. Tablet treatment is sometimes used under specialist supervision in severe cases.

For more severe types of inherited ichthyosis, genetic intervention may be a treatment of the future.

IMPETIGO

A bacterial infection characterized by "weeping" blisters.

What are the symptoms?

Small blisters appear on a background of red skin. These burst, releasing pus, which dries to form honey-colored crusts. Local lymph nodes may be enlarged and tender. It is most often seen on the exposed skin of children and is very contagious in this age group. The presence of infection can be confirmed by the doctor taking a culture.

What are the treatment options?

Affected children should be kept out of school until the area starts to heal, and towels should not be shared. Very mild cases may clear up simply with regular cleaning. If a few small areas are affected, antibiotic cream should be used for 7 to 10 days. For more extensive cases, oral antibiotics are used in combination with cream for a 7-day period.

Most episodes will clear up with the above measures. If not, a swab is necessary to check for unusual bacteria, and the possibility of reinfection from an untreated source should be considered. Impetigo may develop into the more severe condition of cellulitis (p. 137) if not treated effectively.

ITCH
Itch is the most common symptom of skin disease.

The term "itch" is used to describe the sensation that makes us want to scratch. The mechanism of itch is poorly understood, and a variety of chemicals are thought to be involved. One of the most important is histamine, which is contained in mast cells found in the skin. Antihistamines are used to relieve itch in skin conditions such as eczema.

Expectation plays a part in itch. Hearing someone talk about bugs and insects, for example, can set off a desire to scratch even though there is no actual physical stimulation of the skin. Itch may also be caused by diseases of the skin or the internal organs, as a side effect of drugs or because of excessive drying of the skin.

There is no specific cure for itch. Scratching is thought to relieve itch by sending a stronger signal to the brain, thus overwhelming the weaker impulse that caused the itch.

KELOID
Keloid scarring is an exaggerated or overgrown response to injury, although it may also occur spontaneously in undamaged skin.

What are the symptoms?
Raised reddish purple or flesh-colored scars, which may extend beyond the boundaries of the original wound are typical. Keloids are most often seen on the chest, neck, back, and shoulders, especially in young adults, although they can appear in older people. They are also more prevalent in people of Afro-Caribbean origin. It is thought that there is an inherited tendency to develop this type of scarring.

What are the treatment options?
Steroids can be used to try to reduce the scars. Steroid cream applied regularly may help, but more often, steroid injected into the keloid is required—small amounts of steroid are injected into the surface of the affected skin. Over repeated injections, the coloring and bulk of the scar may reduce, giving a more acceptable cosmetic appearance. Steroid-impregnated tape, which is available through doctors, can also be applied.

What is the outlook?
After one episode of keloid scarring, it is likely that the problem will recur with future skin damage. Unnecessary operations and procedures should therefore be avoided.

KERATOACANTHOMA
A growth found in sun-exposed parts of the body, particularly in fair-skinned people.

What are the symptoms?
A small papule appears suddenly and grows quickly over a matter of weeks to produce a large nodule, 1 inch in diameter, with a horny plug in the center.

What are the treatment options?
If keratoacanthomas are left alone, they may naturally resolve without any treatment, but this will leave a noticeable scar. Keratoacanthomas are a form of skin cancer. Because of this, they are removed under local anesthetic. Once removed, it is unlikely there will be problems.

KERATOSIS PILARIS
Patches of rough skin.

What are the symptoms?
This is an inherited condition that begins in childhood. Hair follicles fill with horny plugs of dead skin cells, leaving rough skin, often with small red or grayish papules around the hair follicles. The outer thighs and upper arms are most commonly involved, but the face may also be affected.

What are the treatment options?
General measures such as the use of emollient soap substitutes, avoiding showers or baths that are too hot and patting rather than rubbing the skin dry may be helpful. Emollients should be used regularly to moisturize the skin, and those containing urea are particularly recommended. The condition generally becomes less obvious in adult life.

LEG ULCERS
Skin loss developing in discolored or swollen skin.

What are the causes?

The most common types of leg ulcer are venous (70 percent), arterial (10 percent), and those caused by diabetes (5 percent).

Venous leg ulcers are caused by impaired drainage of blood away from the leg and back to the heart. Arterial ulcers result from impaired circulation causing a reduced amount of blood to reach the leg. Ulcers can also be caused by inflammation in the walls of the blood vessels (vasculitis).

What are the symptoms?
Venous ulcers are usually preceded by a heaviness and swelling of the lower leg, which may last for years. The skin can become discolored (red or brown) because of leakage of blood from the damaged blood vessels, and there may be eczema in affected areas. Ulceration is most common around the ankle bones, and ulcers may be single or multiple and vary in size and depth.

Arterial ulcers are more commonly found on the toes, heel, or front of the foot. There may be other evidence of arterial problems such as angina or calf pain on walking.

Vasculitic ulcers start as painful spots, becoming small "punched out" ulcers.

How is it diagnosed?
Blood tests, including a diabetes check, may be performed. Swabs may be taken if infection is suspected. Circulation should be tested to determine the type of ulcer and therefore the most appropriate treatment.

What are the treatment options?
Rest and elevation of the leg are important parts of the treatment for venous ulceration. The main aim is to relieve the swelling, and pressure bandaging is very effective (although not to be used in arterial ulceration, as this may worsen the circulation further). The bandages may be changed several times a week depending on the state of the ulcer. Any infection is treated with antibiotic cream or tablets. Varicose vein surgery may help by improving the venous drainage of the leg. For arterial ulcers, surgery may be necessary to improve the circulation. In vasculitic ulcers, the aim is to treat the underlying cause.

What is the outlook?
Healing is a slow process and can take years; some ulcers never heal. Once varicose ulcers have healed, compression stockings should be worn daily to try to prevent recurrence.

ON THE CUTTING EDGE

The eradication of leprosy

In 1991, the World Health Organization launched its target of eliminating leprosy as a global health problem by 2000 through

- Ensuring that all health centers had adequate stocks of multidrug treatment (MDT).
- Education campaigns to encourage people with "suspicious" skin markings to seek treatment.
- Health education to ensure that patients took all medications regularly and completely.
- Keeping accurate records to monitor progress.

Elimination was defined as less than 1 new case per 10,000 population, and the target was met. Despite the global reduction in cases, however, leprosy remains a significant problem in six countries: Brazil, Madagascar, India, Myanmar, Nepal, and Mozambique. Efforts are now being aimed at reducing the prevalence of the disease in those countries and repeating the global success at the local level in those areas and regions where leprosy is still common—largely sub-Saharan and central Africa and Indonesia.

LEPROSY
Also known as Hansen's disease, after the Norwegian doctor who discovered the responsible bacteria.

Leprosy is caused by infection with a type of bacterium similar to the one that causes tuberculosis. It is spread by droplet infection and close contact, much like the flu, and although not found naturally in the United States, it remains an important problem in parts of Asia and Africa. Well-defined areas of altered pigment appear and are numb, leading to an increased risk of injury. There may be ulceration of the skin, and some areas become thickened, particularly on the face. A biopsy of the skin and nerves confirms the diagnosis. Treatment—in the form of dapsone in combination with oral antituberculous drugs—may be required for life.

LICHEN PLANUS
A common, sometimes chronic, skin disorder.

Males and females are affected equally by this condition, which occurs most often in middle age. Shiny, purple, flat-topped papules appear on the skin in varying sizes, often with clusters round the wrists, ankles, and genitalia. The papules can also be seen in areas of skin damage (the appearance of a skin condition in areas of broken or damaged skin is known as the Koebner phenomenon). The lesions are often itchy, although they may cause no symptoms. In 50 percent of cases, the mucous membranes (lining of the mouth, genital area) are involved, and these areas may be affected alone. In 10 percent of cases the fingernails are affected, causing grooving and ridging of the nail. A similar appearance can be caused by some prescribed drugs, so a skin biopsy may be performed to confirm the diagnosis.

What are the treatment options?
Treatment can only control symptoms—it is not curative and takes the form of steroid cream or ointment applied twice daily when itchy. If the condition is very severe or widespread, steroid tablets may be prescribed, and a steroid paste or spray can be used for painful mouth lesions.

Lichen planus tends to clear up on its own over a period of 3 months to 2 years, although affected areas may appear darker than usual for some months afterwards (this is known as postinflammatory hyperpigmentation). If the mouth is affected, this can take decades to resolve, and there is a very small risk of developing localized skin cancer within the mouth. Phototherapy (p. 112) may be used for stubborn itch. Less than 20 percent of sufferers will have a further attack in their lifetime.

LICHEN SCLEROSUS ET ATROPHICUS
An inflammatory disease mainly affecting middle-aged to elderly women, although it may occur in children.

What are the symptoms?
This condition usually targets the genital area, causing itching, painful intercourse, and pain with passing urine, although it may be asymptomatic. The skin of the labia and clitoris appears white, shiny, and thinning, and there may be loss of the normal structure in more advanced cases. It less often affects skin at virtually any other body site. There is a male equivalent, involving the penis, known as balanitis xerotica obliterans.

How is it diagnosed?
Diagnosis is generally made by appearance, although a biopsy can be helpful and is essential in areas not responding to treatment. Other conditions such as allergic skin disease may need to be excluded.

What are the treatment options?
Treatment consists of using a soap substitute for washing combined with a strong steroid cream regularly initially and then used as needed. In advanced cases, removal of the foreskin in men will take out affected skin; surgery in women and children is an option once the condition is under control and scarred or damaged skin can be excised. This condition can progress to skin cancer, although this is rare and can take many years. It is important to notify a doctor of any areas that are changing or unresponsive to treatment.

LICHEN SIMPLEX
Also known as neurodermatitis, this skin problem is partly self-inflicted.

Lichen simplex is caused by repeated rubbing or scratching of a certain area of skin either out of habit or as a manifestation of stress. There is not necessarily any underlying skin complaint. The skin becomes red and thickened with obvious creases. The back of the neck, lower legs, and anal-genital area are common sites to be affected, and biopsy is only necessary if the diagnosis is in doubt. Steroid creams combined with covering of the affected area may help to break the habit and affected sites will clear up with treatment. However, patches do tend to recur either in the same site or elsewhere.

LUPUS ERYTHEMATOSUS
A multisystem autoimmune disorder that may be limited in some cases to the skin.

What are the causes?
Lupus is caused by the body producing antibodies against itself. It may affect the skin alone or other body systems, too. Any internal organ may be affected. It is more common in females and in the Black and Chinese populations.

What are the symptoms?
The rash seen in lupus consists of scaly red plaques, often in sun-exposed sites, although any area may be affected. Redness of the cheeks and nose is common. The lesions may clear up to leave scarring, and alopecia may be a feature.

How is it diagnosed?
No single test exists to diagnose lupus. If it is suspected, blood and urine testing and a skin biopsy are necessary to determine the type and extent of involvement.

What are the treatment options?

Sunlight aggravates the skin condition in lupus in 25 percent of patients, and should be avoided with the use of high-factor sunscreen and sun-protective clothing. Strong steroid creams are used on the rash, and these may be combined with steroid tablets in more severe cases. Antimalarial drugs are helpful in extensive cases, and these, along with other treatments, may be prescribed by a specialist.

There is no cure for lupus; the aim is to control symptoms. Many cases of skin-restricted lupus resolve spontaneously.

LYME DISEASE

Named after Lyme, Connecticut, where the disease was first recognized, this condition results from a tick bite.

This condition is caused by the microorganism *Borrelia burgdorferi*, which is transmitted by the bite of a tick. Not everyone affected recalls being bitten, but after about a week, a slowly expanding red circular patch forms around the bite. In some cases, the infection may spread to other areas of the body and may cause joint pains, irregularities of the heartbeat, and nervous system problems. Diagnosis can be confirmed by a blood test. If only the skin is involved, oral antibiotics are used; intravenous antibiotics are necessary if any spread of infection has occurred. Antibiotics should cure the skin infection. However, if the disease has spread, cure is not always guaranteed even with intensive treatment.

MALIGNANT MELANOMA

The least common, but potentially fatal, skin cancer.

What are the causes?

Sunburn, particularly in childhood, plays a major role in the development of this cancer. Having an immediate family member who has had melanoma increases the risk, as does the presence of multiple moles. Females are more commonly affected than males, and the incidence is rapidly increasing.

What are the symptoms?

Although melanomas often occur in normal skin, when they appear like a "new" mole, one in three arises in an existing mole. Any of the following changes in a mole should be checked:

• asymmetry
• border irregularity
• color irregularity

Other changes to note are inflammation, crusting, itching, or bleeding. A mole on any part of the body, including fingernails, toenails, and soles, can be affected.

Scotland has the highest rate of malignant melanoma in the UK. Researchers are unsure whether this is because of the higher numbers of people with Celtic (fair-skinned) coloring.

How is it diagnosed?

A full examination is necessary. If melanoma is suspected, the affected area should be removed. Blood tests and X-rays may be performed, depending on the extent of the tumor. Chemotherapy, radiation, surgery, or immunotherapy may be used in more advanced cases.

What is the outlook?

The prognosis depends on the thickness of the melanoma; for thin melanomas, the outlook is excellent. Diagnosis at an early stage is therefore important. Regular follow-up appointments are essential after removal to check the original site and the rest of the skin for suspicious areas.

MILIA

Milia—tiny white spots on the skin—are very common.

Milia may occur on areas of damaged skin or in sweat ducts or sebaceous glands as white cysts and especially on the face. They occur at any age and are most common in young women. No treatment is necessary, but the overlying skin can be pierced with the tip of a sterile needle and the cyst removed, if so desired. Milia are likely to go away without treatment, although many are removed for cosmetic reasons.

MOLES AND PIGMENTATION

Areas of pigmented and often raised skin.

The average white-skinned adult may have up to 50 moles. The presence of more than this number is a risk factor for developing malignant melanoma, so individuals with a large number should cover up and take extra care in the sun.

ACQUIRED MELANOCYTIC NEVUS

This is the most common type of mole, which is roughly .08 to .12 inch in diameter, with a regular color. These usually appear from early childhood. No treatment is required unless there is concern about possible malignant change, in which case they can be surgically removed.

ATYPICAL NEVI

These may have an irregular edge or color or may be inflamed. Increased numbers may be found in people with melanoma. Suspicious examples should be removed. If they are present in large numbers, the doctor will usually recommend referral to a hospital for regular photography and monitoring.

CONGENITAL NEVI

These are present from birth and found in about 1 percent of all babies. They can vary in size from a tenth of an inch to covering a large area of the body, although this is rare.

FRECKLES

Freckles are caused by an increased production of pigment in localized areas in the skin. These are stimulated by the sun to give the very common flat light-brown macules. They are especially common in fair-haired people and redheads and indicate a sensitivity to the sun.

HALO NEVUS

This is seen most commonly on the backs of teenagers and is so called because there is a circle of paler skin around the mole, which will often fade completely. This is caused by immunological attack on the mole, which is destroyed, with some loss of surrounding pigment cells. The pale skin is prone to burning, so it should be protected in the sun.

LIVER SPOTS

These flat brown macules are common on sun-exposed sites from middle age. They have a regular color and distinct edge and may be treated with cryotherapy (p. 119). Malignant change is possible over many years, so any change in color or size should be reported to your doctor.

MELASMA/CHLOASMA

This is an increase in pigment production caused by hormonal changes and is commonly seen on the faces of pregnant women or those on the contraceptive pill. Sunlight darkens the pigment, so use of a sunscreen is recommended.

MOLLUSCUM CONTAGIOSUM
Small skin lesions, commonly seen in children.

This is caused by viral infection and affects mainly children. It is spread by direct contact, through sharing towels for example, with shiny whitish-pink nodules with a small pit in the middle appearing 2 to 6 weeks after contact. They can affect any area of the body. Multiple lesions are common, and they may be particularly numerous in children with eczema. Although generally without symptoms, they can become inflamed. An iodine-based paint can be prescribed for inflamed areas (but this is not commonly used); the condition generally resolves without treatment. Recovery may take up to 18 months, and the condition does not recur.

MYCOSIS FUNGOIDES
A low-grade cancer of the immune system, which also involves the skin.

What are the symptoms?

Mycosis fungoides affects less than 1 in 100,000 of the population, commonly middle-aged adults. Its cause is unknown, although genetic, environmental, and viral triggers may all play a part. Red scaly patches appear, especially in covered sites such as the buttocks, trunk, upper inner arms, and thighs. This progresses to plaques, then skin tumors, and it may eventually affect other systems in the body. The whole process may take many years. The patches may be itchy or asymptomatic. It can be difficult to differentiate between the early lesions and the much more common conditions of eczema and psoriasis. In the later stages, hair loss and enlarged lymph nodes may be present.

How is it diagnosed?

Diagnosis is made by skin biopsy, although this can be inconclusive in the early stages and may need to be repeated over a number of years. In later stages, blood tests can help indicate if spread to other areas has taken place.

What are the treatment options?

Follow-up is necessary to assess the stage and to look for evidence of internal spread. In the precancerous stages, symptoms may be controlled by the regular use of emollients and topical steroids. Phototherapy (p. 112) can relieve symptoms and also lead to remission. However, the majority of cases relapse when treatment stops. Radiation or chemotherapy is used in later stages.

What is the outlook?

The outlook can be good: Most individuals with the condition die in old age from other causes. In a few cases, however, advanced disease may be reached in 2 to 3 years.

NECROBIOSIS LIPOIDICA
Painless plaques on the fronts of the shins.

Necrobiosis lipoidica is associated with diabetes, although less than 1 percent of diabetics are affected. It also appears in nondiabetics or before diabetes has been diagnosed.
It is characterized by shiny, waxy yellow or red plaques with easily visible blood vessels. These are not usually sore or itchy but may ulcerate and be difficult to heal. Diagnosis is made on appearance, although biopsy can be helpful if there is any doubt. Diabetes should be tested for if not already known to be present. This condition is typically persistent and difficult to treat, although steroid creams may be tried and cosmetics can be used to cover the affected areas.

NEUROFIBROMATOSIS
Multiple abnormalities of soft tissue and nerves.

What are the causes?
This genetically determined disease affects 1 in 3000 of the population, although 50 percent have no affected family member and the cause is a new gene mutation. There are two types: Type 1 is known as Von Recklinghausen's disease and affects the skin; type 2 affects the nervous system.

What are the symptoms?
Multiple neurofibromas are seen. These are soft, flesh-colored, dome-shaped nodules a tenth of an inch to a little over an inch in diameter. Typically, they feel as if they can be pushed inward, as if through a buttonhole. Other features include the presence of freckles in the axillary (armpit) area, and at least six light brown patches (known as café-au-lait patches) appear before one year of age. However, neurofibromas tend not to be seen until puberty and increase in number throughout life.

What are the treatment options?
If neurofibromatosis is suspected, hospital referral is needed for confirmation and further management. Large neurofibromas can be removed if they are a nuisance. Hospital follow-up is recommended, and confirmed cases should receive genetic counseling regarding future family.

What is the outlook?
There is a small risk of neurofibromas becoming malignant. In the future, DNA screening prior to conception may help identify those at risk. Children of affected adults have a 1 in 2 chance of developing the disease.

PAPULAR URTICARIA
The manifestation of an allergic reaction to insect bites.

Itchy papules—especially on the arms and legs, but often distributed asymmetrically across the body—tend to occur in groups and clear up leaving a small scar or area of increased coloring. The spots can become infected from scratching. Diagnosis is usually made on examination. It can be confirmed by identifying the cause. Pets should be examined by a vet. Grooming pets over a plastic sheet will catch any bugs they may be harboring, and these can then be taken to the vet for analysis.

Anti-itch creams or calamine lotion can be used to relieve the symptoms, as can antihistamines, but the main treatment is to eradicate the cause: Insect repellents may be needed.

PARONYCHIA
An infection in the skin surrounding the fingernails and toenails.

Paronychia may be acute—lasting a few days or so—caused by bacteria entering through damaged skin or the cuticle. The nail fold is tender and swollen, and pus may be produced. There is also a chronic version that may be caused by a combination of bacteria and yeast organisms. In chronic paronychia, the nail can be ridged and discolored. Chronic paronychia is more common in people with diabetes, with poor circulation, with recurrent yeast infections, and in those who do wet work or work with flour.

Any pus produced should be swabbed and tested. Testing for diabetes and yeast infection may be necessary. Oral antibiotics or antifungals in combination with antifungal cream are used depending on the identified cause. Over-manicuring of the cuticles should be stopped, and the hands should be kept warm and dry. Acute paronychias generally settle with antibiotics, although occasionally they need to be lanced to release a buildup of pus.

PEMPHIGOID/PEMPHIGUS
Conditions in which the skin blisters and separates.

These two conditions are autoimmune disorders: Antibodies that attack some of the proteins that hold the layers of the skin together are produced by the body, leading to separation and blister formation. In pemphigus, the blisters form near the skin surface; in pemphigoid, the problem is deeper.

Pemiphigoid tends to affect the elderly. Blisters may arise anywhere and can be very itchy. Pemphigus sufferers tend to be younger and may be more unwell. It is a severe condition—potentially fatal in extreme cases. Blisters may appear first in the mouth, making eating painful, and spread to the face, back, chest, and scalp. The blisters rupture easily.

Diagnosis is confirmed by biopsy, and blood tests may be performed to test for antibodies in the circulation. Strong steroid creams are used in combination with steroid tablets. Hospital admission may be necessary for pemphigus. Steroids may be required for several months in a gradually reducing dose. However, the natural progression is for these conditions to burn out over a period of months to years.

PILONIDAL SINUS
A condition in which one or more hairs ingrow into the skin of the cleft of the buttocks, causing inflammation and often leading to abscess formation.

The condition affects more men than women and is rare after age 40. It can cause and may produce a discharge. Antibiotics may be of some benefit, but often surgery to remove the hair, drain the abscess, and then close the skin is the only effective treatment. This can often be treated on an outpatient basis, using sedation and local anesthetic.

PITYRIASIS ROSEA
An often otherwise asymptomatic red rash.

Pityriasis rosea is most common in young adults and children, especially in the spring and autumn. It starts as a single, 1 to 2 inch diameter red patch, which is followed about a week later by crops of similar lesions with a fine scale on the chest, abdomen, back, and upper arms. The lesions on the back may be lined up along the skin creases giving a "Christmas tree" appearance. The rash is usually asymptomatic but may be itchy. Although the cause has not been confirmed, it may be viral. It is not caused by a fungus, bacteria, or an allergy.

Like some viral diseases, pityriasis rosea usually occurs only once. Unlike many viruses, however, pityriasis rosea does not seem to be contagious.

This condition is benign and usually resolves in 4 to 8 weeks, with no recurrence. Moisturizers and anti-itch creams may be used if necessary. Sunlight may hasten recovery.

PITYRIASIS VERSICOLOR
A mild fungal infection causing changes in pigment.

This noninfectious condition is caused by overgrowth of yeasts, which normally live on the skin, in response to hot, humid conditions. Acids released by the yeasts cause alteration in skin pigmentation. Young adults are most commonly affected, with pale brown or pinkish oval papules appearing on the trunk. In the sun, these areas do not tan.

Skin scrapings reveal the responsible yeasts. Antifungal creams can be applied at night for several weeks, in combination with the use of antifungal shampoo twice a week, using the lather to wash the body. Oral antifungal tablets may also be taken. Untreated areas will persist, but treated areas will return to normal. Recurrences are common.

POLYMORPHIC LIGHT ERUPTION
A condition that results from being in the sun.

Itchy red plaques, papules, and vesicles appear in exposed areas within 24 hours of sun exposure. Females are more commonly affected, and there may be a history of the condition in the family. The rash appears in spring and persists through the summer but improves as a tan develops. It tends to recur annually.

The regular use of sunscreen and sun-protective clothing may be sufficient to control the condition in mild cases. Weak steroid cream can be used to clear up the rash. Desensitization treatment is commonly used: A short course of phototherapy (p. 112) is given in the spring to "harden" the skin to the effects of the sun and give a mild protective tan. Light testing can be performed in hospitals to look for an exaggerated response to controlled amounts.

PORPHYRIA
A multisystem metabolic disorder, which in the past may have triggered some of the myths surrounding werewolves, because its symptoms include a low tolerance of sunlight and excessive growth of body hair.

The porphyrias are a group of rare, inherited disorders in which an enzyme is lacking, leading to a build-up of proteins in the bloodstream. These proteins, known as porphyrins, are toxic to the nervous system and cause increased sensitivity to sunlight. The skin becomes fragile and may develop red blisters, especially on the face and back of the hands. Scarring and increased hair growth may occur in these sites.

Porphyrins can be tested for by a specialist. The porphyrin level is treated and kept down by regular removal of a proportion of the blood from the circulation. Sunscreens are necessary, and antimalarial drugs may be helpful. There is no cure at present for some of the porphyrias, although in time gene therapy may be possible. Some types may be cured simply by removal of triggering factors, such as alcohol and some medications.

PSORIASIS
A chronic scaling skin disorder, often hereditary.

What are the causes?
The cause of psoriasis is not completely understood, but there is a hereditary component, with 80 percent of psoriasis caused by genetic factors. The underlying problem is a more rapid life cycle of the cells that make up the epidermis. In susceptible individuals, psoriasis may be triggered by factors such as infection or drugs (such as beta-blockers); it is then made worse by factors such as stress or alcohol.

What are the symptoms?
Psoriasis may develop at any age. It typically consists of well-demarcated red plaques with a silvery scaly surface. The knees and elbows are common sites, but any area may be affected. The scalp is often involved, with thick scales appearing, and the nails may have multiple small pits. Scars or areas of injury tend to be a focus for psoriasis (known as the Koebner phenomenon), and arthritis may also be a feature.

More than 7 million Americans suffer from psoriasis. It generally appears between ages 15 and 35, but about 13 percent of new cases every year are in children under 10.

Guttate psoriasis is a particular type that follows throat infections in children and young adults. The psoriasis plaques are smaller (like rain drops) and tend to resolve with no treatment within about 2 months. A minority of sufferers may go on to develop psoriasis in adult life.

How is it diagnosed?
Diagnosis is made from the appearance of the condition. Skin lesions and nails may be mistaken for fungal infection, in which case skin scrapings and nail clippings will be analyzed.

What are the treatment options?
There is no cure for psoriasis; the aim of treatment is to control and suppress symptoms and try to delay flare-ups.

Moisturizers should be used to reduce scaling. A variety of creams including coal tar, steroids, and vitamin D–based creams can be used on the plaques. Coal tar can be messy, but the newer preparations are easier and cleaner to use. Strong steroids, although effective, may cause a rebound to worsen when stopped. Vitamin D–based creams increase maturation of the cells and modulate the immune response, causing the disorder and should be the treatment of choice. They may be used with steroids to counteract inflammation.

Sunlight or phototherapy (p. 112) is an effective treatment for most people and may provide relief for several months or longer. For severe cases, cytotoxic tablets may be prescribed, although these all have potential side effects, so regular blood tests are necessary. Shampoos are available for scalp psoriasis, and if necessary the scale can be softened with olive oil or proprietary creams prior to shampooing out. Nail psoriasis is hard to treat, but it may improve with oral treatments.

What is the outlook?
Psoriasis is a life-long condition, but it is possible to go for long periods with no symptoms. It is important not to let the treatment become more of a nuisance than the condition. If one parent has psoriasis, his or her child has a 25–30 percent chance of having the condition. This increases to 60 percent if both parents are affected.

PYODERMA GANGRENOSUM
Ulcers caused by rapid inflammation of the skin.

This is often found in conjunction with other conditions, such as inflammatory bowel disease, arthritis, or vasculitis (p. 154). The cause is not fully understood, but it may be caused by an abnormal reaction by the immune system. Ulcers develop either singly or in crops, most commonly on the lower legs. These may start as a pustule or nodule with surrounding redness, which rapidly extends to give an ulcer with a distinct, reddish-purple edge. They are painful, and there may be associated fever with general aches and pains. Diagnosis is made from appearance and biopsy. Depending on other symptoms, more tests may be needed to look for associated conditions. The ulcers will require a dressing and rest and elevation to encourage healing. Oral steroids are used to control the condition and prevent further spread. It may take months for pyoderma gangrenosum to clear, but treatment of any associated condition may hasten recovery.

PYOGENIC GRANULOMA
A small fleshy vascular nodule formed in response to trauma, commonly on the hands or feet.

Pyogenic granulomas develop within days or weeks in sites of trauma, such as a prick by a needle or thorn, although the incident is not always remembered. The surface of the nodule is fragile and tends to bleed easily when hit. Diagnosis is usually clear to a doctor from appearance. However, because certain skin cancers can share this appearance, the removed tissue is always analysed. The nodule may reduce without treatment, but because of inconvenience and bleeding, surgical removal may be recommended.

ROSACEA
A disorder causing chronic inflammation of the face.

What are the causes?
The cause is unknown, but inherited susceptibility is likely to play a part. Demodex mites, which are naturally present in hair follicles and associated sebaceous glands, are found in larger numbers in rosacea sufferers, but it is unlikely that they are involved in its evolution. Certain food, such as tea, coffee, chocolate, cheese, alcohol, curry, vinegar, and citrus fruits may aggravate the condition, but patients should never be put on an exclusion diet without identifying the exacerbating agents for themselves. It can also be worsened by sun, wind, cold, heat, and cigarette smoke. Steroid creams and ointments can also exacerbate it.

What are the symptoms?
Rosacea affects approximately 1 percent of 30 to 60 year olds, although it may be seen from the early teens on. Women are commonly affected, although it is often more severe in men.

In the early stages, flushing (which is more intense than normal blushing) is the most common feature. The flushing episodes become more prolonged, until a fixed redness of the face develops, affecting the nose, cheeks, chin, and forehead. Papules and pustules then develop in the sites of redness, and in more severe cases, the skin can become unevenly thickened (for example, in rhinophyma, swelling of the nose, which may be mistaken as being related to alcohol). The skin is typically more irritable and sensitive, and in 50 percent of sufferers, the eyes will also be affected (ocular rosacea). The diagnosis is generally made with clinical appearance and history.

What are the treatment options?
There is no cure for rosacea, but in most patients, it is self-limiting. A variety of treatments can be used to control the symptoms. Use of oil-free and fragrance-free skincare products is beneficial, and a soap substitute is less irritating for washing. Green-tinted foundation can counteract the red appearance. The avoidance of triggering factors and regular use of a sunscreen (at least SPF 20) can also help.

If these simple measures are not sufficient, antibiotic gels or creams can be prescribed in combination with antibiotic tablets, if necessary. Antibiotics are taken in full dose for 2 to 3 weeks, then reduced according to symptoms. Flushing or redness can be treated using drugs with specific effects on blood vessels. With successful treatment, the papules and pustules tend to reduce first, but the reddening takes longer to respond. Antibiotic treatment may be required for months or years. Severe cases of rosacea may need referral to a dermatologist for alternative treatments, including surgery for rhinophyma and laser treatment to reduce facial redness.

Although the condition does tend to resolve in time, it may persist for anything from a year to several decades.

SCABIES
The skin's response to infestation by a mite.

What are the causes?
Scabies is caused by the mite *Sarcoptes scabei*. It is transferred from person to person through close body contact, although 4 to 6 weeks can elapse between contact and the development of symptoms.

What are the symptoms?
The main feature of scabies is itch, which is worse at night. Itchy papules are seen on the wrists, hands, nipples, umbilical area, and genitals, with little "burrows" between the fingers. There may be an associated eczema-type rash affecting the skin from the neck downward.

How is it diagnosed?
The diagnosis is usually evident, with a typical body rash and a history of contact with an affected person. If in doubt, a doctor may open a burrow with the tip of a needle to see if a mite can be extracted.

What are the treatment options?
The affected person, all family or household members, and any close contacts should be treated at the same time, whether

itching or not. Cream can be obtained from the doctor, and it is essential to follow the instructions fully. It is applied to the whole body from the neck down prior to going to bed. If hands are washed during the night, the cream must be reapplied. The length of application depends on the preparation used. After treatment, all bed linen and clothes should be laundered.

What is the outlook?
The itch may persist for up to a week after treatment, even if treatment was successful. However, if new spots are still appearing a week later, the treatment must be repeated, perhaps using an alternative preparation.

SEBACEOUS CYST
A benign growth under the skin.

Sebaceous cysts form when the release of sebum from the skin is blocked. They are smooth to the touch, range in size, and occur most commonly on the scalp, face, ears, and genitals. They only require treatment if they become infected and painful or are excessively large. See p. 138.

SEBORRHEIC DERMATITIS
A type of eczema often only on the scalp but sometimes on the face, throat, underarm, and groin.

What are the causes?
Seborrheic dermatitis is common, with males more often affected than females. The condition is common in adults aged 30 to 60 and in babies up to the age of 3 months. Affected babies do not necessarily develop the condition in adult life. Originally, seborrheic dermatitis was simply thought to be caused by increased sebum production from the sebaceous glands, but it now seems likely that other factors are implicated. *Pityrosporum ovale*, a yeast normally found on the skin, is present in increased numbers, and climate may also play a part—improvement is often seen in spring and summer. The condition can worsen with stress.

What are the symptoms?
In infants, the most common manifestation is cradle cap, in which yellow-brown, greasy scales adhere to the scalp skin. Scaling may also be evident on the eyebrows, forehead, temple, and behind the ears. The diaper area becomes red and scaly, with a clearly defined edge. Infants are generally not distressed by this condition.

In adults, the scaliness may be confined to the scalp, where it is seen as dandruff. However, it may be more widespread, affecting the face, behind the ears, eyelids, chest, and back. The groin area and skin under the breasts are also commonly affected. Affected skin is generally red, scaly, and crusty, and additional infection with yeasts or bacteria is common in both the infant and adult forms.

What are the treatment options?
In infants, the regular use of emollients both as a soap substitute and moisturizer is recommended, including to the diaper area. A mild steroid cream combined with an antifungal agent can be used on affected areas if necessary. Frequent shampooing is helpful in lifting the scales on the scalp, and an olive oil scalp massage a couple of hours before shampooing can improve the results.

For adults, frequent use of an antiyeast shampoo with vigorous massage is helpful, using the lather from the shampoo to wash the body. Steroid creams combined with an anti-infective agent are often used. In widespread or stubborn cases, antifungal tablets may be required.

Infants tend to recover by the age of one, but the condition may be chronic in adults, with fluctuations in severity.

SEBORRHEIC KERATOSES
An extremely common benign skin condition, also known as a seborrheic wart.

Typically these are greasy, brown lesions with a warty surface that look as if they have been stuck onto the skin, but the color can vary from pink to black. They are seen mainly after 40 years of age, and any site can be affected. Some people may have one or two, but others have dozens in varying sizes. The cause is unknown: Genetics, viral infection, or sun exposure may play a part. No treatment is necessary because these are benign, not infectious, and have no effect on health. However, they may be unsightly or catch on clothing, in which case they can be frozen with liquid nitrogen (p. 119). Particularly large warts can be removed under local anesthetic if necessary.

SHINGLES (HERPES ZOSTER)
Shingles is caused by the chicken pox virus.

After a bout of chicken pox, the virus remains dormant in the nerves and may reactivate at any time to cause shingles, which begins as a burning pain in the skin. This is followed by a crop of blisters that burst and crust along the path of the nerve. In mild cases, rest and painkillers may be all that is required. Antiviral tablets can be given but are only effective if started within 48 hours of the rash appearing. Shingles is self-limiting, but ongoing pain after the rash has cleared may be a problem. Shingles is contagious: Someone who has not had chicken pox may develop it after exposure to shingles.

SQUAMOUS CELL CARCINOMA (SCC)
The second most common type of skin cancer.

What are the causes?
The main cause of SCC is excessive sun exposure. It is more common in outdoor workers and those with outdoor hobbies, especially if they are fair-skinned. Impairment of the immune system, whether by disease or medication, also increases the likelihood of SCC. The average age of onset is 60 to 65 years.

What are the symptoms?
SCCs occur in sites that are exposed to the sun (face, ears, the back of the hands). They tend to start as warty nodules or plaques (see actinic keratoses, p. 134) and may thicken and become sore as they grow. The surface is red and crusty and may bleed or ulcerate. They grow steadily and measure from a tenth of an inch to a little over an inch in diameter. Diagnosis is usually suggested by the appearance and confirmed by biopsy or after removal.

What are the treatment options?
The main treatment is surgical removal under anesthetic. Radiation is also sometimes used. It is important to avoid excess sun, so wearing a hat and long sleeves and using SPF 20 or higher sunscreen when outdoors are necessary.

What is the outlook?
Although spread to other areas of the body is rare, there is an increased chance of spread if the cancer affects the lips or ears. Therefore, anyone affected by SCC needs regular checkups to ensure the skin remains clear and there is no sign of spread. Most people with SCC are completely cured.

URTICARIA
An itchy red rash, also known as hives or nettle rash.

What are the causes?
Urticaria can be caused by a wide range of triggers, including sunlight, cold, pressure, exercise, heat, certain medications, and certain foods. It may also indicate an underlying disease. In most cases, there is no identifiable cause.

What are the symptoms?
Itchy red plaques, papules, or weals with a white center suddenly arise, often within minutes. Each one may last up to 24 hours then fade without trace. In some cases, swelling of the skin round the eyes and mouth is also seen.

How is it diagnosed?
Biopsy is not generally necessary, because diagnosis can usually be made from the appearance and history. Blood and urine testing plus X-rays may be performed if an underlying illness is suspected.

What are the treatment options?
Any known trigger should be avoided or removed, if possible. Aspirin, codeine, and any aspirin-based medicines should also be avoided: These are known to worsen urticaria.

Antihistamine tablets should be taken regularly in urticaria of unknown cause. Severe cases may need steroid tablets or referral to a doctor if not clearing up.

What is the outlook?
Urticaria caused by a certain trigger will clear up when the cause is removed. Most people will heal over a few months.

VASCULITIS
Inflammation of the blood vessels in the skin or internally.

Vasculitis may be triggered by infection, illness, or medication, or it can be of unknown cause. The lower legs are commonly affected, with painful, purplish spots. If larger blood vessels are affected, the skin ulcerates, and there may be a feeling of malaise if internal blood vessels are affected. A biopsy will confirm skin lesion diagnosis. Blood tests, X-rays, and urine analysis may be performed to look for illness. Triggering factors need to be identified and dealt with. In mild cases, no treatment may be necessary; however, in more severe cases rest is important, and oral steroids may be given.

VITILIGO
A cause of loss of skin pigment.

What are the causes?
Vitiligo affects approximately 1 person in 100 and is caused by a loss of melanocytes in the skin. This is caused

by an autoimmune disease in which the body attacks its own melanocytes. Other autoimmune diseases, such as thyroid disease, diabetes, and pernicious anemia, may be associated. In 30 percent of cases, there is a history of affected family members. All races can be affected.

What are the symptoms?
White areas of skin with a distinct edge appear, especially around the eyes, mouth, genital region, hands, wrists, and knees, and often in a symmetrical pattern. It occurs most commonly in the 20s, although any age group can be affected. It may be seen first in sites of injury or sunburn. Diagnosis is generally self-evident.

What are the treatment options?
Vitiligo can be a difficult condition to treat successfully, and the outlook is unpredictable, because the affected areas may remain static, spread, or, rarely, repigment. Cosmetics can be used to camouflage the paler areas, and steroid or vitamin D creams may be beneficial. Phototherapy (p. 112) is effective in some cases, although months of treatment may be necessary, and any benefits may be lost when treatment ends. Sunscreen should be used to protect the depigmented area.

WARTS
Warts are caused by the human papilloma virus.

Warts are spread by direct contact with someone who has warts or via shed patches of skin, for example in swimming pools. It can take a few weeks to several months to develop warts after being in contact with the virus. Planters warts are a form of wart that affects the feet.

What are the symptoms?
The most common type of wart is a firm papule with a rough surface ranging in size from a tenth to half an inch in diameter. These are usually found on the hands. Planters warts are often found in groups on the feet.

   Flat warts are seen mainly on the face and can be difficult to treat. Warts affecting the anal or genital region should be seen by a doctor.

How is it diagnosed?
Warts are obvious, but in older people they may be mistaken for more serious problems. If there is doubt, the surface can be scraped to reveal "black dots"—tiny blood vessels.

What are the treatment options?
Treatment is not essential. Most warts go away eventually if left alone. However, most people prefer to treat warts. Creams are available without prescription. Before application, the wart should be soaked and then gently rubbed with a pumice stone or emery board. After drying, the cream is applied to the wart and covered with a bandage. This should be repeated daily. If there is no benefit in 12 weeks, a doctor may offer cryotherapy (p. 119).

Warts are rare in babies, common in children, and peak at 16 to 18 years of age, when 20 percent of young people have at least one.

What is the outlook?
With treatment, 99 percent of warts will eventually disappear. Even with no treatment, it is normal for warts to resolve, although this can take anyhere from 3 months to 3 years.

XANTHELASMA/XANTHOMA
Raised yellowish papules and plaques on the skin.

These soft yellowish plaques/papules appear round the eyes (xanthelasma) or other body sites (xanthoma) and are caused by deposits of fatty material in the skin. The majority of xanthelasmas are of cosmetic concern only, whereas xanthomas are more likely to be associated with elevated fat and cholesterol levels in the blood. Although diagnosis is clear from their appearance, blood tests should be performed to look for raised cholesterol levels, which may need treatment: The skin lesions usually do not cause problems, but can be treated with trichloracetic acid.

XERODERMA PIGMENTOSUM
The inability of the body to repair sun damage.

This rare genetic disease causes an increased sensitivity to sunlight from infancy, associated with premature aging of the skin and the development of skin cancers. Strict sun avoidance is essential and skin cancers must be removed as they occur. Oral treatment may reduce the risk of cancer development. In some cases, lifespan is shortened, but the disease varies greatly in severity.

Index

Acknowledgments

Carroll & Brown Limited would also like to thank:

Picture researcher
Sandra Schneider

Production manager
Karol Davies

Production controller
Nigel Reed

Computer management
Paul Stradling

Indexer
Jill Dormon

3-D anatomy
Mirashade/Matt Gould

Illustrators
Andy Baker, Rajeev Doshi/Regraphica, Kevin Jones Associates, Mikki Rain, John Woodcock

Layout and illustration assistance
Joanna Cameron

Photographers
Jules Selmes, David Yems

Photographic sources
SPL = Science Photo Library

6   *(right)* Getty Images
7   Eye of Science/SPL
8   *(top left)* SPL
10 *(top)* Neil Bromhall/SPL
    (bottom right) Getty Images
11 *(center)* Sheila Terry/SPL
    (right) Dr. P. Marazzi/SPL
    (bottom) SPL
12 Gavriel Jecan/Corbis
13 H. Raguet/Eurelios/SPL
28 Getty Images
30 Professors P. M. Motta, K. R. Porter & P. M. Andrews/SPL
33 *(left)* Alfred Pasieka/SPL
    (right) Daniel Sambraus/SPL
34 *(top right)* Ken Bank/RetnaUK
34–35 Getty Images
36 Getty Images
36–37 Michael Keller/Corbis
38 *(center)* Getty Images
    (right) Getty Images
39 Getty Images

40 *(left)* Getty Images
    (top right) Getty Images
    (3rd from top) Getty Images
    (4th from top) Getty Images
    (5th from top) Getty Images
43 Getty Images
44 Getty Images
45 Getty Images
46 *(bottom left)* Getty Images/ Eyewire
47 *(center, right)* Getty Images
48 Getty Images
49 Getty Images
51 Getty Images
53 Getty Images
55 Getty Images
59 *(top)* Getty Images
60 Getty Images
61 Ellipse Pulsed Light Ltd, 45-47 Cheval Place, London SW7 1EW www.3d.dk
62 Getty Images
70 Getty Images
73 *(top right)* Getty Images/Eyewire
    (bottom right) Getty Images
74 Getty Images
76 Getty Images
77 *(background, top, top right)* Getty Images
    (bottom) Advanced Safety Devices www.safety-devices.com
78 *(top)* Getty Images
    (center) Peter Scoones/SPL
    (bottom) Getty Images/Eyewire
79 Getty Images
80 Getty Images/Eyewire
81 Getty Images
82 Getty Images
83 *(top right, 3rd from top)* Getty Images
84 *(left, center right, right)* Getty Images
85 T. H. Foto-Werbung/SPL
87 Getty Images
92 Getty Images
93 Melle Stripp www.allthingsnails.co.uk
94 Getty Images
100 *(left)* Saturn Stills/SPL
    (center) Dr. Arthur Tucker/SPL
    (right) Eye of Science/SPL
101 David Parker/SPL
104 Dr. A. Chu
107 *(top)* Dr. A. Chu
    (bottom) Dr. P. Marazzi/SPL
108 John Durham/SPL
109 St. John's Institute of Dermatology

110 *(top)* Saturn Stills/SPL
    (bottom) SPL
111 David Parker/SPL
112 St. John's Institute of Dermatology
113 Jim Selby/SPL
116 Eye of Science/SPL
117 *(top)* Eye of Science/SPL
    (bottom) SPL
118 Getty Images
119 AntoniaReeve/SPL
120 Dr. Chris Hale/SPL
121 Dr. P. Marazzi/SPL
122 Mike Devlin/SPL
123 James Stevenson/SPL
124 *(top)* Dr. P. Marazzi/SPL
    (bottom) Tony McConnell/SPL
125 Belle Santé UK Ltd www.beauty-guild.co.uk
126 BSIP Laurent H. Americain/SPL
127 Wellcome Trust Medical Photographic Library
128 Dr. Brian Coghlan
129 Dr. Brian Coghlan
130 Dr. Arthur Tucker/SPL
131 *(top)* Dr. P. Marazzi/SPL
    (center) SimonFraser/NCCT, Freeman Trust, Newcastle-upon-Tyne/SPL
    (bottom) Dr. P. Marazzi/SPL
132 *(top)* James Stevenson/SPL
    (bottom) Nancy Kedersha/ Immunogen/SPL

Back cover *(right)* Jim Selby/SPL

Contact details
National Institutes of Health
http://www.nih.gov

American Society of Plastic Surgeons
http://www.plasticsurgery.org

American Association of Tissue Banks
http://www.aatb.org

619–009–1